SURGERY – PROCEDURES, COMPLICATIONS, AND RESULTS

LIVER STEATOSIS AND BARIATRIC SURGERY

Surgery – Procedures, Complications, and Results

Additional books and e-books in this series can be found on Nova's website under the Series tab.

SURGERY – PROCEDURES, COMPLICATIONS, AND RESULTS

LIVER STEATOSIS AND BARIATRIC SURGERY

JAIME RUIZ-TOVAR
AND
LOREA ZUBIAGA
EDITORS

nova
Medicine & Health
New York

Library of Congress Cataloging-in-Publication Data

ISBN: 978-1-53616-444-2
Library of Congress Control Number:2019950991

Published by Nova Science Publishers, Inc. † New York

CONTENTS

PREFACE

Obesity is actually considered as a pandemia in developed countries. Some authors have even described it as the "pandemia of the 21st century". The reality is that obesity rates are increasing in Western countries and, even in developing countries, this begins to be a real problem.

Although we are living in a society based on the image of the person, based on the concept that a good image is associated with success (professional and personal success), obesity is not only an image problem, but it is a health problem. Obesity is associated with many metabolic disorders, such as diabetes mellitus, dyslipidemia, hypertension, sleep apnea-hypopnea syndrome, ... Far away from the psychological impact, obesity and its related comorbidities are silent diseases. These are mostly asymptomatic for long time, and it is just when the symptoms appear, that the damage is already irreversible. The objective of the fight against obesity is to prevent the appearance of these permanent damages, increasing then the life expectative and the quality of life.

For morbidly obese patients, bariatric surgery is the best option to achieve a significant and maintained weight loss. Moreover, surgical treatment is the best method to obtain a significant improvement and even remission of most obesity-related comorbidities. When analyzing the evolution of comorbidities after bariatric surgery, most studies focus on the effects on diabetes mellitus, hypertension and dyslipidemia. Non-alcoholic fatty liver disease (NAFLD) is gaining importance as obesity-related comorbidity, as the prevalence of NAFLD at any degree can reach up to 95% of morbidly obese patients. Liver steatosis is the mildest expression of NAFLD, but nearly 25% of bariatric patients can present Non-alcoholic steatohepatitis (NASH) and in up to 2% of the cases the liver affection might develop to cirrhosis.

Bariatric surgery has demonstrated to improve NAFLD, obtaining a remission in up to 90% of the cases, depending on the approach performed and in many cases the remission depends on the preoperative liver damage rather than on the weight loss obtained.

Actually, there is increasing evidence that the liver status must be careful evaluated before surgery and monitored postoperatively and even the liver damage is also a criterium to consider when electing the most appropriate bariatric approach for a patient.

We hope that this book, based on the current evidence of NAFLD in obese patients, the diagnostic methods available and the effects of bariatric surgery, can be helpful in the routine clinical practice. However, we must keep always in mine, that scientific knowledge is continuously advancing, and actual evidence can be outdated next year, requiring future updates.

Finally, we want to thank to all the contributing authors, all of them friends and experts in their corresponding fields, their availability, time and efforts to write all the chapters included in the book.

Jaime Ruiz-Tovar, MD, PhD
Lorea Zubiaga, MD, PhD
Editors

In: Liver Steatosis and Bariatric Surgery
Editors: Jaime Ruiz-Tovar et al.
ISBN: 978-1-53616-444-2

Chapter 1

INTRODUCTION TO NAFLD AND NASH : ETIOPATHOGENESIS

Soledad García-Gómez-Heras, MD, PhD,
Julio Paredes-González and Raquel Franco-Rodríguez
Human Histology and Pathology, Health Science Department,
Rey Juan Carlos University, Madrid, Spain

ABSTRACT

The liver, a principal metabolic organ, is the target of metabolic disorders which may lead to the development of non-alcoholic fatty liver disease (NAFLD) and non-alcoholic steatohepatitis (NASH). NAFLD and NASH represent different stages of the same disease, and appear to be multifactorial. Etiopathogenesis is complex and currently the underlying mechanisms are not completely understood; there have been different hypotheses describing the pathogenesis; the main three are: the "two hits," "three hits," and "multiple hits" hypotheses. Here, we explain all the factors that seem to influence the development and the outcome of this disease.

Keywords: liver-histology, NASH/NADFL etiopathogenesis, two-hits hypotheses, three- hits hypotheses, multiple-hits hypotheses

INTRODUCTION

The liver, a principal metabolic organ, is frequently the target of various metabolic disorders, which may lead to the development of non-alcoholic fatty liver disease (NAFLD) and non-alcoholic steatohepatitis (NASH). These conditions are associated with obesity and insulin resistance, and they are considered a hepatic manifestation of the Metabolic Syndrome (MS).

Also, liver disease can lead to systemic metabolic abnormalities. NAFLD/NASH is an emerging risk factor for obesity, dyslipidemia, type 2 diabetes, cardiovascular disease, and chronic kidney disease.

The term NAFLD includes a spectrum of fatty liver diseases ranging from simple steatosis to NASH and cirrhosis.

NAFLD is defined as an accumulation of fat in the hepatocytes when excessive drinking of alcohol or any other secondary cause is not present.

NAFLD is considered benign and reversible. Patients who suffer only hepatic steatosis may have a good prognosis in the long term, 10–20% develop NASH, defined as steatosis with hepatic inflammation, hepatocyte injury with or without fibrosis. NASH can progress to more severe stages such as cirrhosis and hepatocellular carcinoma (HCC).

Currently, NAFLD/NASH is one of the most prevalent chronic liver diseases, and is emerging as a global public health threat

THE LIVER

The liver is both an exocrine and endocrine gland, located at the "crossroad" of the digestive tract and the rest of the organism. Some of the main functions of an adult liver include:

- bile production, as the main exocrine function,
- conservation of metabolic balance,
- glycogen storage,
- drug degradation,
- toxin degradation,
- plasma protein synthesis,
- vitamins (A, D and K) processing, and storage,
- iron storage, metabolism, and homeostasis,
- immunoglobulin A secretion,
- secretion of growth actors.

Therefore, the scope of liver disease consequences is large, due to the dependence of other organs on the liver's metabolic functions.

In the embryo, in the 4th week of gestation, the liver starts developing from the hepatic diverticulum, which is an endodermal evagination of the anterior primitive intestine.

Adult liver cells proceed from different embryonic origins:

- the liver bud arises from the anterior intestine, giving place to hepatocytes and the choledocus epithelial lining.
- umbilical and vitelline veins are the origin of vascular sinusoids.
- from the septum transversum: stroma and hepatic capsule, hematopoietic cells, Kupffer cells, smooth muscle, and connective tissue of bile ducts.

During the fetal period, the liver has a double role: bile synthesis (from the 12th week) and hematopoiesis. From the first gestational weeks, groups of hematopoietic cells appear between hepatocytes and the blood vessel walls. The liver assumes its role as hematopoietic organ from the third month to the seventh month of gestation, when such function begins to decrease and the bone marrow becomes the main hematopoietic organ, thus causing liver volume to decrease from 10% of body volume in a 10-gestational week embryo to less than 5% of total body volume in a full-term fetus.

Anatomically, in an adult, the liver is coated with Glisson's capsule, a fibrous connective tissue capsule, and the visceral peritoneum, a serous cover.

Macroscopically, it is divided into four lobes: right, left, quadrate, and caudate lobe or Spiegel's lobe. Such division is only important topographically. The division in functional or surgical segments, based on blood supply and biliary drainage, is more important.

In order to understand the liver's functions and pathology, its vascularization should be described.

Liver Vascularization

This organ presents double irrigation: the portal vein and the hepatic artery (branch of the celiac trunk). They both access through the hepatic hilum. The liver receives blood that has previously irrigated the intestine, the spleen and the pancreas, and thus contains:

- nutritional and toxic substances proceeding from the intestine
- erythrocyte and erythrocyte degradation products from the spleen
- endocrine secretions from the pancreas
- enteroendocrine cell secretions from the digestive tract

The liver is interposed in the course of the blood vessels transporting the substances absorbed in the digestive tract. It is the first organ receiving metabolic substrates and nutritional substances. But it is also exposed to toxic components that may have been absorbed.

Around 75% of irrigation proceeds from the portal vein that carries venous blood that has poor oxygen concentration. Since the blood from the two sources is mixed just before perfusing the hepatocytes, they are never fully exposed to oxygenated blood.

Inside the liver, distribution branches of the portal vein and the hepatic artery deliver blood to sinusoid capillaries which will irrigate the hepatocytes. Branches of the portal vein, arteries, and biliary drainage (which disgorge in a common hepatic duct) flow jointly and create the "portal triad."

Sinusoid capillaries flow in close contact with hepatocytes, disgorge into a central or centrolobular vein, which in turn drains into supralobular veins. The blood leaves the liver through suprahepatic veins, which disgorge in the inferior vena cava.

HISTOLOGICAL ORGANIZATION OF THE LIVER

The liver is formed by the parenchyma, which consists of trabeculae or chords of hepatocytes that are organized in only one cell of thickness in adults. These chords are separated by sinusoid blood capillaries with a lumen of around a 15 micron diameter. The wall is formed by a single layer of endothelial cells with a large number of fenestrations and surrounded by a discontinuous basal membrane. Such organization allows for direct contact among the substances circulating in the blood and the cells forming and surrounding capillaries.

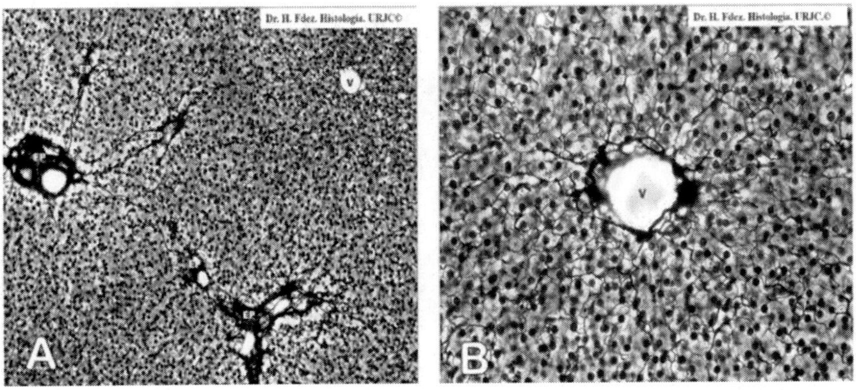

Figure 1. Human Liver. The stroma of liver is constituted by a reticular connective tissue with collagen III, impregnated in black with silver carbonate. As seen in the image A, these fibers increase their proportion in the portal spaces(ES). V: centrilobular vein. Del Rio Ortega Silver Carbonate Technique. 50x. In image B, we can observe in more detail the reinforcement of collagen III around the centrilobular vein. Ortega Silver Carbonate Technique. 200x.

The stroma is a connective tissue connected with the fibrous capsule of Glisson. Blood vessels, lymph vessels, nervous branches, and bile ducts can be found in it. In the connective tissue of the narrow space between hepatocytes and sinusoid capillaries, reticular fibers (or type III fibers) are predominant, whereas collagen I is predominant in portal spaces (Figure 1).

Liver Lobules

There are three possible histological models to describe the structure of the liver: classic lobule, portal lobule, and liver acinus (Figure 2).

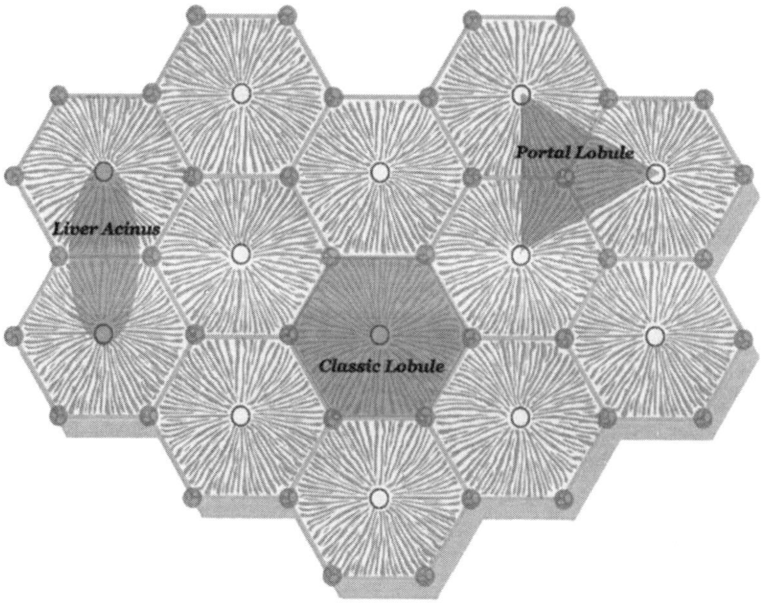

Figure 2. Scheme with the three types of liver lobules.

Classic Lobule

This is the classical and easiest-to-see mode to consider hepatic organization. It is based on the distribution of the portal vein and the hepatic artery branches inside the organ, and the route followed by the blood coming from these vessels when it perfuses the hepatocytes.

In a hepatic classic lobule, cuts present a more or less hexagonal tissue mass. Each lobule measures 0.2 x 0.7 mm. It is composed of one-cell-thick plates of anastomosed hepatic trabeculae, separated by liver sinusoids. There is a vein at the center, the post-sinusoidal hepatic venule, referred to as the central vein or centrilobular vein, in which sinusoids discharge.

Hepatocyte plates and the corresponding sinusoids have a radial disposition from the centrilobular vein towards the periphery of the lobule. In the hexagon angles, there are the portal spaces with triads surrounded by loose connective tissue, which is continuous with the Glisson fibrous capsule.

Portal Lobule

Exocrine liver functions stand out, particularly in bile secretion. Therefore, the morphological axis is the interlobular bile duct of the portal triad of the classic lobule.

The external edges are the imaginary lines mapped out connecting the three centrilobular veins that lay closest to that portal triad. These lines define a tissular region similar to a triangle, which includes those portions of the three classic lobules that secrete bile. Bile is drained in the axial bile duct (Figure 3).

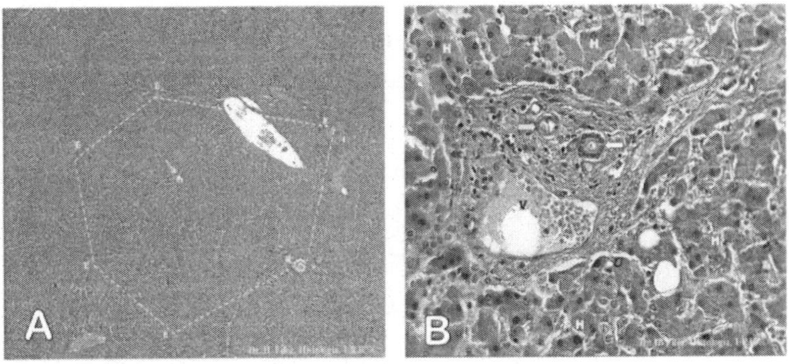

Figure 3. A. Histological image of a human liver, being complicated the delimitation of the lobules (dashed line). We can appreciate the presence of a centrilobular vein (arrow) and portal space around it (E). Hematoxylin-Eosin, 100x. B. Here we can observe a portal space of a human liver. Within the dashed line, portal space and its structures: vein(V), artery (yellow arrow) and bile duct (white arrow). H: liver parenchyma. Hematoxylin-Eosin. 250X.

Liver Acinus

This is the structural unit that best groups and coordinates blood perfusion, metabolic activity, and hepatic pathology. This structure allows for a description of the liver's exocrine function.

The acinus has a rhomboid shape. The minor axis is defined by the terminal branches of the portal triad, which coincide with the limits of two classic lobules, and the main axis is a perpendicular line drawn between the two centrilobular veins closer to the minor axis. Therefore, in a two-dimensional view, the liver acinus occupies part of two contiguous classic lobules.

Based on this organization, hepatocytes in each acinus are described as lying in three concentric elliptical zones that surround the short axis:

- zone 1: closest to the short axis and the irrigation coming from the portal vein and the hepatic artery branches. This zone corresponds to the periphery of classic lobules.
- zone 3: the most distant to the short axis and the closest to the centrilobular vein. This zone corresponds to the center of the classic lobule, whose hepatocytes surround the centrilobular vein.
- zone 2: between zone 1 and 3, but with no clear limits.

The division of hepatic parenchyma in zones is indispensable for the description and interpretation of the hepatic lesion distribution due to ischemia, or to exposition to toxic substances, in order to assess the level of tissue degeneration and cell regeneration in every clinical situation.

Due to the sinusoidal blood flow, the oxygen gradient, metabolic activity of hepatocytes and hepatic enzyme distribution vary in the three zones.

Zone 1 cells are the first to receive oxygen, nutrients and toxins from the sinusoidal blood. Thus, they are the first to exhibit morphological alterations after a bile duct obstruction. These cells are also the last to die if there are circulation disorders, and the first to regenerate.

Zone 2 cells have morphological and functional characteristics, as well as responses, that are intermediate between cells in Zones 1 and 3.

Zone 3 cells are the first to suffer ischemic necrosis (centrilobular necrosis) in situations where perfusion is altered, and the first to accumulate lipids. They are the last to respond to toxic substances and biliary stasis.

In Zones 1 and 3, normal variations of enzymatic activity, the amount and dimensions of cytoplasmic organelles, and the size of glycogen cell deposits can be confirmed.

Liver Cells

Hepatocytes

They represent 80% of the parenchyma (Figure 4). They are big polyhedral cells, measuring around 20 x 30 microns. Their big nuclei are located in the cell center, and several are binucleated. The mean life of these cells is relatively long, around 5 months, and they have a huge capacity to regenerate.

200 to 300 *peroxisomes* can be found in the cytoplasm of each cell. Their function is similar to that of mitochondria, and they are a site of important oxygen consumption. A large number of oxidases (which generate hydrogen peroxide), catalases (enzymes degradating hydrogen peroxide to oxygen and water), D-amino acid oxidase, and alcohol dehydrogenase can be found in them. Peroxisomes intervene in the degradation of fatty acids (through beta-oxidation), in glycogenesis, and in purine metabolism. They also participate in the detox processes that take place in the liver, such as alcohol detox.

The *Smooth Endoplasmic Reticulum* (SER) of hepatocytes can be very extensive, but it will depend on the functional moment. It contains enzymes that participate in the degradation and conjugation of toxins and drugs, cholesterol synthesis enzymes, and enzymes of lipoproteins lipid component. In overburdened liver conditions, due to drugs or hormones, the synthesis of new SER membranes and their associated enzymes is induced. Hypertrophy is also experienced after the administration of alcohol, drugs (phenobarbital, anabolic steroids and progesterone) and certain chemotherapy agents.

Likewise, the *Golgi apparatus* in these cells is very developed with up to 50 dictyosomes, each composed of 3-5 piled cisterns.

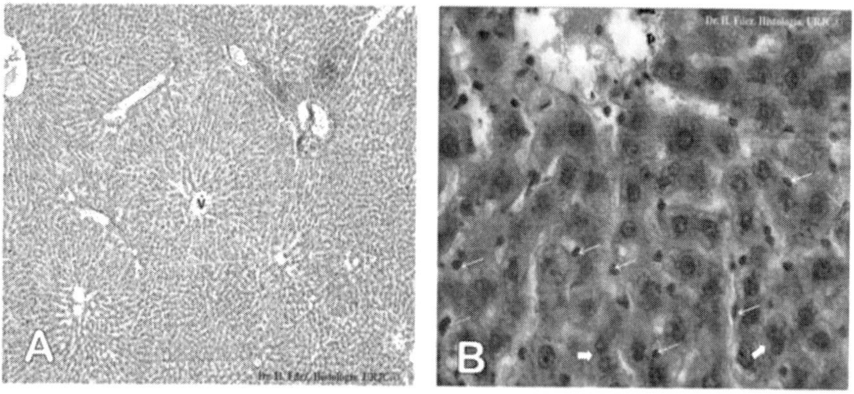

Figure 4. A. Human liver lobule (dashed line). With this histological technique, the stored glycogen in the hepatocytes is highlighted, colored in clear carmine. Carmín de Best Technique. 50 X. B. High-magnification image of the previous preparation. The sinusoids, the hepatocyte cords, as well as the nuclei of the sinusoidal cells (thin white arrows), the Ito cells (yellow arrows) and the Kupffer cells (green arrows) are observed. Carmín de Best Technique. 400 X.

Lysosomes in hepatocytes concentrate close to the bile canaliculus. They can also be a site for normal storing of ferritin, and a ferric accumulation site in certain diseases, due to an excessive deposition.

Macrophages Present in the Liver

Macrophages belong to the phagocytic mononuclear system. Hepatic macrophages consist of resident macrophages called Kupffer cells (KCs) and macrophages that arise from bone marrow-derived monocytes after a stimulus.

KCs lean on the endothelium, and their extensions cross the whole sinusoidal lumen. These are common cells in the endothelial lining of sinusoids, where they create a barrier. They present abundant lysosomes, phagocyte particles and microorganisms that arrive in the hepatic lobules through the blood.

They participate in the final degradation of certain aged or damaged erythrocytes. Erythrocyte and iron fragments, in the form of ferritin, can be observed in their cytoplasm.

They represent a cell of innate immunity. KCs are the body's primary line of defense against microorganisms. Their location is optimal for carrying out their functions inside the liver. During liver injury, KCs initiate the immunological response by rapidly secreting cytokines and chemokines, which induce the recruitment of other immune cells, including monocytes, into the liver. Both populations of macrophages produce proinflammatory and anti-inflammatory cytokines, contributing to chronic inflammation such as that seen in alcoholic liver disease, NAFLD, NASH and other pathological conditions affecting the liver.

Perisinusoidal Space or Space of Disse

This is a zone for intercellular exchange of substances between the blood and hepatocytes. It is defined as the space between the basal surfaces of hepatocytes and the basal surfaces of endothelial cells and Kupffer cells that line the sinusoids. Because of the large gaps in the endothelial layer and the absence of the continuous basal lamina, no significant barrier exists between the blood plasma in the sinusoid and the hepatocyte plasma membrane.

Because of the broad fenestrations between endothelial cells and the discontinuity in the basal membrane, there is no physical barrier between sinusoid blood and the plasma membranes of hepatocytes. Proteins and lipoproteins synthesized by hepatocytes are directly transferred into the blood through this space. This pathway is for liver secretions other than bile.

Ito Cells (or Stellate Cells)

They can also be found in these spaces. Their origin is mesenchymal, and they are the primary storage site for hepatic vitamin A. In certain liver diseases, chronic inflammation, or cirrhosis, Ito cells lose their ability to store lipids and vitamin A, and they differentiate into cells with characteristics of myofibroblasts, with capacity to synthesize collagen. These cells seem to play an important role in hepatic fibrogenesis. They synthesize and deposit collagen I and II in the portal space, as well as in the connective zone surrounding the centrilobular vein.

An increase in perisinusoidal fibrous stroma is an early sign of liver response to toxic substances.

The cytoplasm of cells contains elements of the contractile apparatus, such as α-actin filaments or desmin intermediate filaments. In situations where contraction of these cells is stimulated, the vascular resistance will be empowered within the sinusoids due to their lumen reduction, leading to portal hypertension. Furthermore, Ito cells participate in extracellular matrix remodeling during recovery from liver injury.

In the fetal liver, islands of hematopoietic cells appear in this space. In cases of chronic anemia in the adult, hematopoietic cells may reappear.

Beyond all that has been explained in this section, the fact that the liver depends on a huge functional reserve remains to be highlighted, and in almost all diseases, except for those causing death, regeneration takes place. After resection of 75% of the liver, there is a small hepatic deterioration, and regeneration restores the liver mass in few weeks. When a massive hepatocellular necrosis occurs, but the connective tissue weft remains intact and the patient survives the metabolic aggression of liver failure, tissue restoration may be almost perfect.

ETIOPATHOGENESIS

Etiopathogenesis is complex and currently the underlying mechanisms are not completely understood; NAFLD and NASH represent different stages of the same disease, and appear to be multifactorial. They occur in response to a chronic inflammatory liver state accompanying obesity, insulin resistance, hepatic steatosis, and oxidative stress. The most progressive forms of NAFLD have been related to metabolic syndrome (ME) and obesity. Both liver parenchymal and nonparenchymal cells are affected.

There have been different hypotheses describing the pathogenesis of NAFLD/NASH. The main three are: the "two hits," "three hits," and "multiple hits" hypotheses.

The classical pathogenetic pathway, originally proposed in 1998, was described as the "two hits hypothesis." This theory stated that damage to the liver tissue begins through aberrant triglyceride accumulation, *the first hit,* which induces *the second hit,* the activation of inflammatory mediators, lipotoxic metabolite-induced mitochondrial dysfunction and oxidative stress. These aggressions lead to steatohepatitis and fibrosis.

The "three hits" theory involves inadequate hepatocyte proliferation after cell death triggered by aberrant lipid accumulation and excessive oxidative stress.

Finally, the "multiple hits" hypothesis involves organ-organ interactions in NASH; inflammatory mediators released from adipose tissue and the liver/gut axis are implicated in NASH pathogenesis. In this model, environmental, metabolic and genetic factors contribute to the development and progression of NASH by affecting diverse organs such as the liver, intestines, and adipose tissue. More specifically, excess caloric or inappropriate intake (environmental factor) increases toxic free fatty acid (FFA) and lipid metabolites (lysophosphatidylcholine (LPC), cholesterol and ceramide) in hepatocytes, leading to hepatic steatosis and hepatocyte sublethal/lethal injuries. Subsequently, hepatocyte-derived cytokines/ chemokines and damage-associated molecular patterns (DAMPs) stimulate Kupffer cells (KC) (which promote inflammatory response) and hepatic stellate cells (HSC) (stimulate fibrotic response); this leads to the development of inflammation and fibrosis in the liver. Free fatty acid (FFA) and lipid metabolites derived from diets or synthesized *de novo* also activate KC and HSC. In addition, insulin resistance and obesity (metabolic factor) influence organ crosstalk between the intestine/adipose tissue and the liver, contributing to the development and progression of NASH.

Various studies suggest that variations in several genes related to hepatic lipid metabolism are associated with increased hepatic steatosis in human NAFLD subjects (PNPLA3 (patatin-like phospholipase domain-containing protein 3), TM6SP2 (transmembrane 6 superfamily member 2), and FADS (fatty acid desaturase)). Factors influencing NAFLD and NASH, and collaborating in their development are discussed next.

Lipid Accumulation in the Hepatocytes

In NAFLD, cell lipid accumulation and the subsequent steatosis may result from several mechanisms: excess fat ingestion, increased fat synthesis, decreased fat export and decreased fat oxidation.

Sedentary lifestyle, too caloric diets or inappropriate intake as diets with high glucose, high fructose, high fat or high cholesterol are environmental factors associated with hepatic steatosis and NAFLD/NASH.

In the case of excess dietary glucose or fructose, they enter the liver through the bloodstream after uptake in the small intestine and are subsequently utilized for the production of hepatic triacylglycerol (TG) via de novo fatty acid synthesis, and become a source of hepatic glycogen storage. When there is excessive free fatty acid (FFA) accumulation within hepatocytes generate toxic lipid metabolites and cause hepatocyte injury, consequently, initiation of NASH.

Lipid metabolites such as palmitic acid, lysophosphatidylcholine (LPC), ceramide, and free cholesterol are considered mediators of hepatocellular lipotoxicity and they contribute to the development and progression of NASH. High concentrations are found in the livers of human subjects with NASH.

Palmitic acid has been reported to trigger oxidative stress, endoplasmic reticulum and mitochondrial stresses, causing lipotoxicity and cell death.

LPC generated from palmitic acid triggers mitochondria-dependent apoptotic machinery.

Ceramide synthesized from palmitic acid also causes mitochondrial impairment of the mitochondrial respiratory chain and increases mitochondrial membrane permeability leading to hepatocyte cell death.

Free cholesterol can induce hepatocyte necrosis/apoptosis by depleting mitochondrial glutathione, and can induce hepatocyte necrosis by generating cholesterol crystals within lipid droplets.

Endoplasmic Reticulum (ER) Stress

Endoplasmic reticulum (ER) Stress is associated with the development of NAFL and progression to NASH through direct cell injury and indirect changes in cell signaling pathways.

In situations of hyperinsulinemia and hiperlipidemia, ER stress causes inflammation, apoptosis, and mitochondrial dysfunction.

Increased dietary intake of FFA, *de novo* lipogenesis and adipose lipolysis, together with impaired FFA oxidation, causes an increase in the flux of FFAs within hepatocytes.

Excessive lipid accumulation causes hepatocellular lipotoxicity via cellular and organelle oxidative stresses including endoplasmic reticulum (ER) stress and mitochondrial dysfunction, leading to hepatocyte cell death.

Furthermore, *chronic* ER stress increases the production of reactive oxygen species (ROS). ROS induces activation of nuclear factor Iκκ-β/NF-κB, a master regulator in the production of proinflammatory cytokines (IL-1-β, TNF-α and IL-6).

In addition, chronic ER stress results in hepatic lipid accumulation via activation of de novo fatty acid synthesis in a manner dependent on ER stress-sensing pathways suggesting that a vicious cycle between ER stress and hepatic steatosis may promote the development and progression of NAFLD/NASH.

Activation of Inflammatory Mediators

Steatosis is strongly associated with chronic hepatic inflammation. Different immunological mechanisms are implicated in the NAFLD progression: innate immunity, adaptive immunity, NLRP3 inflammasome activation. As evidence, portal inflammatory infiltrates in human NASH livers are characterized by broad inflammatory cell markers: CD68, CD3, CD8, CD4, CD20, neutrophil elastase, matrix metalloproteinase 9 and interleukins.

Innate Immunity in NAFLD/NASH: Kupffer Cells (KC) and Hepatic Stellate Cells (HCS) in NAFLD/NASH

In NAFLD and its evolution to NASH, the innate immune system is activated by different factors and through different pathways. This creates a vicious cycle difficult to break. Hereunder, some of these factors are discussed.

1. In response to excessive lipids, hepatocytes produce chemokines and pro-inflammatory cytokines (TNF-α, IL-6 and IL-1b); they act on non-parenchymal cells such as KCs and HSCs, which contribute to the progression of NASH.
2. Lipotoxic fatty acids such as palmitic acid and ceramide can activate Kupffer cells and subsequently promote the production of pro-inflammatory cytokines such as CCL2 which recruit more peripheral macrophages, CXCL16 to recruit natural killer T cells, and CXCL1/2/8 to recruit neutrophils (TNFa and IL-6)

In this way, Kupffer cells and recruited innate immune cells coordinately aggravate inflammation in the liver.

Moreover, Kupffer cells and infiltrating macrophages produce several cytokines such as TGFβ, Galectin- 3, platelet-derived growth factor, TNF-α and IL-1β that are able to activate quiescent HSCs and increase their proliferation. More specifically, palmitic acid-induced TNF-α and IL-1β in infiltrating macrophages can cause lipid accumulation and insulin resistance in hepatocytes. Macrophages activated by the palmitic acid, by secreting TNF-α and IL-beta, generate lipid accumulation and insulin resistance in hepatocytes.

1. Apoptotic or necrotic hepatic cells trigger signals for NASH promotion. They release inflammatory cytokines, damage-associated molecular patterns (DAMPs), ATP, uric acid or mitochondrial DNA. DAMPs can cause hepatic inflammation and fibrosis by activating KCs and HSCs via paracrine or endocrine actions.

2. Elevated hepatic expression of inflammatory cytokines such as TNF-α, interleukin-6 (IL-6) and interleukin 1-beta (IL-1β), and activated Kupffer cells, start up the Iκκ-β/NF-κB signaling pathway. Both inflammation and Iκκ-β/NF-κB activation promote carcinogenesis and may also play a key role in hepatocellular carcinoma (HCC) development.
3. Finally, activated Kupffer cells, infiltrating macrophages and hepatocytes secrete NLRP3 inflammasome-dependent IL-1β, which plays a crucial role in the progression of NAFLD/NASH.

The Involvement of Adaptive Immunity: Role of Lymphocytes in NASH

The mechanism involved in the initiation of inflammation in NASH pathogenesis is very similar to other organs. In the initial phase, the resident macrophages secrete chemokines, which recruit CD4+/CD8+ T lymphocytes and NKT cells to the tissue, which enhance macrophage activation and proinflammatory mediator release. Both macrophages and lymphocytes represent the most frequent inflammatory infiltrates of NASH livers. It should be stressed that, in human NASH liver biopsy sections, the portal tract infiltrates are dominated by CD8 (+) lymphocytes.

The B cells also play a critical role in NASH pathogenesis. Lipid peroxidation products from phospholipid oxidation interact with B lymphocytes and are one of the sources of antigens able to promote an adaptive immune response in NASH. As evidence, 40%–60% of patients with NASH have circulating antibodies against lipid peroxidation-derived antigens and the high titers of these antibodies are in parallel with increased risk to develop advanced liver fibrosis.

Insulin Resistance (IR) in NAFLD/NASH Development

Metabolic factors such as obesity, dyslipidemia, and IR come together with NAFLD. In individuals with IR who present excess visceral fat, the influx of FFAs to the liver is increased, thus leading to both triglyceride accumulation and direct lipotoxicity.

Hyperinsulinemia or hyperglycemia, a key feature of insulin resistance, increases hepatic de novo fatty acid synthesis.

So, because of IR, there is greater influx of FFAs to the liver: these undergo β-oxidation or esterification with glycerol to form triglycerides. Additionally, FFAs are able to cause toxicity through directly increasing oxidative stress and activating inflammatory pathways.

On the other hand, insulin resistance in adipose tissue impairs the ability of insulin to suppress lipolysis; consequently, FFAs released from adipose tissue are transported into the liver (FFAs from adipose tissue contribute to 60% of hepatic lipid accumulation).

NAFLD also contributes towards a worsening of IR and the cumulative effect generates a vicious cycle of IR and NAFLD worsening each other. Several abnormalities intrinsic to NAFLD impair insulin receptor signaling, especially: FFAs, tumor necrosis factor-alpha (TNF-α), nuclear factor kappa B (NF-κB), ceramide, Jun N-terminal kinase 1 (JNK1), suppressors of cytokine signaling (SOCS) and cytochrome CYP2E1.

Altered Hepatocyte Proliferation and NAFLD/NASH

Dead hepatocytes are normally replaced by replication of mature hepatocytes so normal liver function is maintained.

In NAFLD, high levels of oxidative stress causes disruption to the regenerative process; mature hepatocytes present impairment of their replication process, and when cell death occurs, the hepatic progenitor cells (HPC) proliferate. These cells have the capacity to differentiate into either hepatocytes or cholangiocytes and may be involved in carcinogenesis relating both to hepatocellular carcinoma and to cholangiocarcinoma, which are the final and most severe consequences of this clinical picture.

It is observed that there is a strong association between expansion of HPCs and a ductular reaction in liver biopsy specimens in NASH cases. The extent of ductular reactions strongly correlates with the degree of fibrosis, suggesting that HPC expansion/ductular reaction do play an important role in stimulating progressive periportal fibrosis.

Inter-Organ Crosstalk in NAFLD/NASH

Adipose tissue and the intestines have a very important role in NAFLD and NASH pathogenesis.

Adipose Tissue-Liver Axis and NASH

Obesity and the associated insulin resistance contribute to the hepatic steatosis, NAFLD and NASH. As we previously mentioned, impaired suppression of insulin-mediated lipolysis in adipose tissue leads to hepatic steatosis through increased fatty acid uptake of hepatocytes. In addition, inflammation in adipose tissue affects hepatic inflammation.

Intestine-Liver Axis and NASH

As discussed below, the impairment of this axis is an important causal factor in the pathogenesis of obesity related steatosis, NAFLD/NASH, liver cancer and diverse liver diseases.

Intestinal permeability and increased gut microbial translocation contribute to the inflammatory pathway involved in nonalcoholic steatohepatitis (NASH) development.

Numerous studies have investigated the association between increased intestinal permeability and NASH.

A meta-analysis was performed by Luther J et al. In 2015, in order to confirm that, they compared the rates of increased intestinal permeability in patients with NASH with healthy controls. NASH patients are more likely to have increased intestinal permeability compared with healthy controls.

In mice, an experimental high fat diet, like NAFLD/NASH diets, induces a decrease in Paneth cell area and a lower production of antimicrobial peptides by these cells, reduced Goblet cell number and their mucin secretion, while intestinal permeability is increased. HFD-fed mice are more susceptible to experimental colitis, severe colonic inflammation, accompanied by the expansion of selected pathobionts such as *Atopobium* sp.

Consequently, bacteria or bacterial products are able to reach the liver through the portal vein. In the liver, conserved motifs of bacteria and bacterial products are recognized by receptors of Kupffer cells, infiltrating macrophages, and HSCs. Lipopolysaccharides and bacterial DNA stimulate multiple signaling cascades via interactions with TLR receptors leading to hepatic steatosis, inflammation, and fibrosis in the liver.

Evidence suggests that lipid intermediates derived from the intestine trigger the development of NAFLD/NASH.

One of the pathways is via intestinal hypoxia-inducible factor HIF-2α, which regulates ceramide metabolism by positive expression of *Neu3*, the gene encoding neuraminidase 3. Human-intestine biopsies from individuals with and without obesity revealed that intestinal HIF-2α signaling was positively correlated with body-mass index and hepatic toxicity. This correlation was verified in mice with an intestine-specific disruption of HIF-2α, in which high-fat-diet-induced hepatic steatosis and obesity were substantially lower as compared to control mice. Intestine HIF-2α inhibition with specific inhibitor markedly reduced intestine and serum ceramide levels.

Gut Bacterial Overgrowth in the Pathogenesis of NASH

Gut microbiota analysis revealed that individuals with NAFLD have a lower percentage of Bacteroides with higher levels of Prevotella and Porphyromonas species compared to healthy controls.

Another study found that the inflammasome-mediated dysbiosis of gut microbiota exacerbates hepatic steatosis and inflammation through enhancing liver TNF-α production.

A murine model of high-fat diet–induced (HFD-induced) NAFLD was used. This study demonstrated that gut microbiota influences NAFLD pathogenesis by regulating the bile acid/intestinal FXR (intestinal farnesoid X receptor) axis that alters the ceramide pathway in the liver and, combined with reduced bacterial fermentation in the gut, results in decreased hepatic lipids. Furthermore, this work reveals an essential role for intestinal FXR in controlling liver lipid metabolism and provides a potential therapeutic strategy for the prevention of disease progression in patients with NAFLD.

Hepatic macrophages play a critical role in maintaining immune homeostasis of the liver.

The liver is constantly exposed to antigens and low levels of endotoxins from the gut since 75% of the liver's blood is supplied from the portal vein.

In normal conditions, small amounts of endotoxins from gut bacteria enter the liver and most of them are eliminated by KCs.

However, the altered composition of microbiota, gut permeability increases and hyper-responsibility of KCs to the gut-derived endotoxin can interrupt this tolerance.

M1 macrophages are abundant and play a critical role in driving inflammation and hepatocyte injury. Macrophage M2 activation is initiated by cytokines IL-10 and IL-4 releasing from prolonged ER stressed hepatocytes.

Macrophage in NASH is associated with toll-like receptor TLR4 activation. During liver injury, macrophages release proinflammatory cytokines such as IL-1β, TNF-α, and IL-6 through the activation of TLR4.

When prolonged, this contributes to T cell activation and results in hepatocyte death and subsequent activation of HSCs.

During NASH, liver macrophages engulf an excessive amount of oxidized low-density lipoprotein and form "foam cells." These macrophage-derived foam cells predominantly contain enlarged lysosomes filled with cholesterol and cholesterol crystals. Increased cholesterol storage inside lysosomes of KCs is associated with hepatic inflammation.

References

Albano E., Mottaran E., Vidali M. et al. "Immune response towards lipid peroxidation products as a predictor of progression of non-alcoholic fatty liver disease to advanced fibrosis." *Gut.* 2005. Vol. 54, 7:.987–993.

Arora A. S., Jones B. J., Patel T. C., Bronk S. F., Gores G. J. "Ceramide induces hepatocyte cell death through disruption of mitochondrial function in the rat." *Hepatology*. 1997. Vol. 25:958-63.

Baiceanu A, Mesdom P, Lagouge M, Foufelle F. "Endoplasmic reticulum proteostasis in hepatic steatosis." *Nat Rev Endocrinol.* 2016. Vol 12:710–22.

Bieghs V., Verheyen F., van Gorp P. J. et al. "Internalization of modified lipids by CD36 and SR-A leads to hepatic inflammation and lysosomal cholesterol storage in Kupffer cells," *PLoS ONE*. 2012. Vol. 7, 3, ArticleI De 34378.

Bieghs V., van Gorp P. J., Walenbergh S. M. A. et al. "Specific immunization strategies against oxidized low-density lipoprotein:a novel way to reduce non alcoholic steatohepatitis in mice,." *Hepatology*. 2012. Vol. 56, 3:894–903.

Bijnen M., Josefs T., Cuijpers I., Maalsen C. J., van de Gaar J., Vroomen M., et al. "Adipose tissue macrophages induce hepatic neutrophil recruitment and macrophage accumulation in mice." *Gut*. 2018. Vol. 67:1317-27.

Broz P., Dixit V. M. "Inflammasomes: mechanism of assembly, regulation and signaling." *Nat Rev Immunol*. 2016. Vol. 16:407–20.

Cazzo E., Pareja J. C., Chaim E. A. "Nonalcoholic fatty liver disease and bariatric surgery: a comprehensive review." *Sao Paulo Med J*. 2017. 135 (3):277-295.

Chiappini F., Coilly A., Kadar H., Gual P., Tran A., Desterke C., et al. "Metabolism dysregulation induces a specific lipid signature of nonalcoholic steatohepatitis in patients." *Sci Rep*. 2017. Vol7:46658.

Day C. P and James O. F. W. "Hepatic steatosis: innocent bystander or guilty party?" *Hepatology,* 1998, vol. 27, 6:1463– 1466.

Day C. P. and James O. F. W., "Steatohepatitis: a tale of two 'Hits'?." *Gastroenterology,* 1998. vol. 114, 4I:842–845. (Bis).

Del Campo J. A., Gallego P., Grande L. "Role of inflammatory response in liver diseases: Therapeutic strategies." *World J Hepatol*. 2018. Vol. 10:1–7.

Donnelly K. L., Smith C. I., Schwarzenberg S. J., Jessurun J., Boldt M. D., Parks EJ. "Sources of fatty acids stored in liver and secreted via lipoproteins in patients with nonalcoholic fatty liver disease." *J Clin Invest*. 2005. Vol. 115:1343–51.

Eguchi A., Wree A. and Feldstein A. E. "Biomarkers of liver cell death," *Journal of Hepatology*. 2014. Vol.60, 5:1063–1074.

Eslam M, Valenti L, Romeo S. "Genetics and epigenetics of NAFLD and NASH: clinical impact." *J Hepatol.* 2018. Vol 68:268–79.

Fang D. L., Wan Y., Shen W., Cao J., Sun Z. X., Yu H. H., Zhang Q., Cheng W. H., Chen J., Ning B. "Endoplasmic reticulum stress leads to lipid accumulation through upregulation of SREBP-1c in normal hepatic and hepatoma cells." *Mol Cell Biochem.* 2013. Vol. 381:127–137.

Feldstein A. E., Werneburg N. W., Canbay A., Guicciardi M. E., Bronk S. F., Rydzewski R., et al. "Free fatty acids promote hepatic lipotoxicity by stimulating TNF-alpha expression via a lysosomal pathway." *Hepatology.* 2004. Vol. 40:185-94.

Friedman S. L., "Liverfibrosis in 2013: convergent pathways that cause hepatic fibrosis in NASH." *Nature Reviews Gastroenterology & Hepatology.* 2013. Vol.10, .2: 71–72.

Gadd V. L., Skoien R., Powell E. E. et al. "The portal inflammatory infiltrate and ductular reaction in human non alcoholic fatty liver disease," *Hepatology,* 2014. Vol. 59, 4: 1393–1405.

Han MS, Park SY, Shinzawa K, Kim S, Chung KW, Lee JH, et al. "Lysophosphatidylcholine as a death effector in the lipoapoptosis of hepatocytes." *J Lipid Res.* 2008. Vol. 49:84–97.

Henderson NC, Mackinnon AC, Farnworth SL, Poirier F, Russo FP, Iredale J. P., et al. "Galectin-3 regulates myofibroblast activation and hepatic fibrosis." *Proc Natl Acad Sci USA.* 2006. Vol 103:5060–5.

Henao-Mejia J., Elinav E., Jin C. et al. "Inflammasomemediated dysbiosis regulates progression of NAFLD and obesity." *Nature,* 2012. Vol.482: 179–185.

Hirsova P., Gores G. J. "Death receptor-mediated cell death and proinflammatory signaling in nonalcoholic steatohepatitis." *Cell Mol Gastroenterol Hepatol.* 2015. Vol. 1:17–27.

Hirsova P, Ibrahim SH, Gores GJ, Malhi H. "Lipotoxic lethal and sublethal stress signaling in hepatocytes: relevance to NASH pathogenesis." J *Lipid Res.* 2016. Vol 57:1758–70.

Ibrahim S. H., Hirsova P., Gores G. J. "Non-alcoholic steatohepatitis pathogenesis: sublethal hepatocyte injury as a driver of liver inflammation." *Gut.* 2018. Vol. 67:963–72.

Ioannou G. N., Subramanian S., Chait A., Haigh W. G., Yeh M. M., Farrell G. C., et al. "Cholesterol crystallization within hepatocyte lipid droplets and its role in murine NASH." *J Lipid Res*. 2017. Vol. 58:1067–79.

Jiang C., Xie C., Li F., Zhang L., Nichols R. G., Krausz K. W., et al. "Intestinal farnesoid X receptor signaling promotes nonalcoholic fatty liver disease." *J Clin Invest*. 2015. 125:386–402.

Kim K. H. and Lee M. S." Pathogenesis of Nonalcoholic Steatohepatitis and Hormone-Based Therapeutic Approaches. Pathogenesis and Hormone-Based Therapy of NASH." *Frontiers in Endocrinology*. 2018; 9: 485.

Kolios G., Valatas V. and Kouroumalis E. "Role of Kupffer cells in the pathogenesis of liver disease," *World Journal of Gastroenterology. 2006*. Vol. 12, 46:7413–7420.

Lee J. C., Lee H. Y., Kim T. K., Kim M. S., Park Y. M., Kim J., et al. "Obesogenic diet-induced gut barrier dysfunction and pathobiont expansion aggravate experimental colitis." *PLoS ONE*. 2017.12:e0187515.

Li Z., Berk M., McIntyre T. M., Gores G. J., Feldstein A. E. "The lysosomalmitochondrial axis in free fatty acid-induced hepatic lipotoxicity." *Hepatology*. 2008. Vol. 47:1495-503.

Luther J., Garber J. J., Khalili H., Dave M., Bale S. S., Jindal R., et al. "Hepatic injury in nonalcoholic steatohepatitis contributes to altered intestinal permeability." *Cell Mol Gastroenterol Hepatol*. 2015. Vol. 1:222–32.

Luyckx F. H., Lefebvre P. J., Scheen A. J. Non-alcoholic steatohepatitis: Association with obesity and insulin resistance, and influence of weight loss. *Diabetes Metab*. (2000) 26:98–106.

Magee N., Zou A., and Zhang Yuxia. "Pathogenesis of Nonalcoholic Steatohepatitis: Interactions between Liver Parenchymal and Nonparenchymal Cells." *BioMed Research International*. 2016:5170 402.

Mari M, Caballero F., Colell A., Morales A., Caballeria J., Fernandez A., et al. "Mitochondrial free cholesterol loading sensitizes to TNF- and Fas-mediated steatohepatitis." *Cell Metab*. 2006. Vol. 4:185–98.

Marra F, Svegliati-Baroni G. "Lipotoxicity and the gut-liver axis in NASH pathogenesis." *J Hepatol.* 2018. Vol 68:280–95.

Mota M, Banini BA, Cazanave SC, Sanyal AJ. "Molecular mechanisms of lipotoxicity and glucotoxicity in nonalcoholic fatty liver disease." *Hepatology.* 2016; 65:1049-61.

Mouzaki M., Comelli E. M., Arendt B. M. et al. "Intestinal microbiota in patients with nonalcoholic fatty liver disease," *Hepatology.* 2013. Vol. 58, 1: 120–127.

Nobili V., Parola M., Alisietal A. "Oxidative stress parameters in paediatric non-alcoholic fatty liver disease." *International Journal of Molecular Medicine.* 2010. Vol. 26, .4:471–476.

Peverill W., Powell L. W. and R. Skoien. "Evolving concepts in hepathogenesis of NASH: beyond steatosis and inflammation," 2014. *International Journal of Molecular Sciences.* 2014. Vol. 15, 5:8591–8638).

Pradere J. P., Kluwe J., De Minicis S., Jiao J. J., Gwak G. Y., Dapito D. H., et al. "Hepatic macrophages but not dendritic cells contribute to liver fibrosis by promoting the survival of activated hepatic stellate cells in mice." *Hepatology.* 2013. Vol. 58:1461–73.

Richardson M. M., Jonsson J. R., Powell E. E., et al. "Progressive fibrosis in nonalcoholic steatohepatitis: association with altered regeneration and a ductular reaction" *Gastroenterology.* 2007; 133(1):80-90.

Romeo S, Kozlitina J., Xing C., Pertsemlidis A., Cox D., Pennacchio L. A., et al. "Genetic variation in PNPLA3 confers susceptibility to nonalcoholic fatty liver disease." *Nat Genet.* 2008, 40:1461–5.

Sell H., Habich C. and Eckel J. "Adaptive immunity in obesity and insulin resistance." *Nature Reviews Endocrinology.* 2012. Vol. 8, 12: 709–716).

Song E., Ouyang N., Horbelt M., Antus B., Wang M., Exton M. S. "Influence of alternatively and classically activated macrophages on fibrogenic activities of human fibroblasts." *Cell Immunol.* 2000. Vol. 204:19–28.

Sookoian S, Castano GO, Scian R, et al. "Genetic variation in transmembrane 6 superfamily member 2 and the risk of nonalcoholic fatty liver disease and histological disease severity." *Hepatology*. 2015. Vol 61:515–25.

Steneberg P, Sykaras A. G., Backlund F., Straseviciene J., Soderstrom I., Edlund H. "Hyperinsulinemia enhances hepatic expression of the fatty acid transporter Cd36 and provokes hepatosteatosis and hepatic insulin resistance." *J Biol Chem*. 2015. Vol. 290:19034–43.

Svegliati-Baroni G., De Minicis S., Marzioni M. "Hepatic fibrogenesis in response to chronic liver injury: novel insights on the role of cell-to-cell interaction and transition." *Liver Int*. 2008; 28(8):1052-64.

Sutti S., Jindal A., Locatellietal I., "Adaptive immune responses triggered by oxidative stress contribute to hepatic inflammation in NASH." *Hepatology*. 2014 vol. 59, 3:886–897.

Tang T, Sui Y., Lian M, Li Z., Hua J. "Pro-inflammatory activated Kupffer cells by lipids induce hepatic NKT cells deficiency through activation-induced cell death. *PLoS ONE*. 2013. Vol. 8:e81949.

Tilg H. and Moschen A. R. "Evolution of inflammation in nonalcoholic fatty liver disease: the multiple parallel hits hypothesis." *Hepatology*. 2010, vol. 52, 5:1836–1846.

Tsai E., Lee T. P."Diagnosis and Evaluation of Nonalcoholic Fatty Liver Disease/Nonalcoholic Steatohepatitis, Including Noninvasive Biomarkers and Transient Elastography." *Clin Liver Dis*. 2018; 22, 73-92.

Vargas V, Allende H, Lecube A, et al. "Surgically induced weight loss by gastric bypass improves non-alcoholic fatty liver disease in morbid patients with obesity." *World J Hepatol*. 2012; 4(12):382-8.

Vonghia L., Michielsen P. and. Francque S. "Immunological mechanisms in the pathophysiology of non-alcoholic steatohepatitis." *International Journal of Molecular Sciences*. 2013. Vol. 14 (10): 19867–19890.

Walenbergh S. M. A., Koek G. H., Bieghs V., and Shiri Sverdlov R. "Non-alcoholic steatohepatitis: the role of oxidized low-density lipoproteins," *Journal of Hepatology*, 2013. Vol. 58, 4: 801–810.

Wan J., Benkdane M., Teixeira-Clercetal F. "M2 Kupffer cells promote M1 Kupffer cell apoptosis: a protective mechanism against alcoholic and non-alcoholic fatty liver disease" *Hepatology*. 2014. Vol. 59, 1:130–142.

Wan X., Xu C., Yu C. and Li Y. "Role of NLRP3 inflammasome in the progression of NAFLD to NASH." *Canadian Journal of Gastroenterology and Hepatology*. 2016. Vol.2016.

Wang L., Athinarayanan S., Jiang G., et al. "Fatty acid desaturase 1 gene polymorphisms control human hepatic lipid composition." Hepatology. 2015. Vol 61:119-28.

Wei Y., Wang D., Gentile C. L. Pagliassotti M J. "Reduced endoplasmicreticulum luminal calcium links saturated fatty acid-mediated endoplasmic reticulum stress and cell death in liver cells." *Mol Cell Biochem.* 2009. Vol. 331:31–40.

Wenfeng Z., Yakun W., Di M., Jianping G, Chuanxin W., and H. Chun, "Kupffer cells: increasingly significant role in nonalcoholic fatty liver disease," *Annals of Hepatology*. 2014. Vol. 13, 5: 489–495.

Winer D. A., Winer S., Chng M. H. Y., Shen L., and E. G. Engleman. "B Lymphocytes in obesity-related adipose tissue inflammation and insulin resistance," *Cellular and Molecular Life Sciences*. 2014. Vol. 71, 6:1033–1043.

Xie C, Yagai T, Luo Y, Liang X, Chen T, Wang Q, et al. « Activation of intestinal hypoxia-inducible factor 2alpha during obesity contributes to hepatic steatosis." *Nat Med.* 2017. Vol. 23:1298–308.

Zhan Y. T. and An W., "Roles of liver innate immune cells in nonalcoholic fatty liver disease," *World Journal of Gastroenterology*. 2010, vol. 16, 37, 4652–4660.

Zhang Xue-Qun, Cheng-Fu Xu, Chao-Hui Yu, Wei-Xing Chen, and You-Ming Li. "Role of endoplasmic reticulum stress in the pathogenesis of nonalcoholic fatty liver disease." *World J Gastroenterol*. 2014. Vol. 20(7): 1768–1776.

In: Liver Steatosis and Bariatric Surgery ISBN: 978-1-53616-444-2
Editors: Jaime Ruiz-Tovar et al.

Chapter 2

EPIDEMIOLOGY AND RELEVANCE OF NASH IN PATIENTS WITH MORBID OBESITY

Leire Zarain-Obrador[1], MD
and Manuel Duran-Poveda[1,2,*], MD, PhD
[1]Department of Endocrine and Bariatric Surgery,
King Juan Carlos University Hospital, Madrid, Spain
[2]Department of Surgery, Faculty of Health Sciences,
King Juan Carlos University, Madrid, Spain

ABSTRACT

Obesity, besides being a common risk factor for a wide range of diseases, such as diabetes, cardiovascular disease or cancer, it is associated with an increased risk of developing non-alcoholic fatty liver disease (NAFLD). It also contributes to the progression of different types of liver diseases, including non-alcoholic steatohepatitis (NASH) and even cirrhosis.

The prevalence of NAFLD has risen in the last decades together with obesity and type 2 diabetes mellitus, becoming the most common chronic liver disease worldwide.

* Corresponding Author's Email: manuel.duran@hospitalreyjuancarlos.es.

The treatment of NAFLD is based on weight loss, which can be achieved by lifestyle modifications, pharmacologic therapy or bariatric surgery.

Keywords: non-alcoholic fatty liver disease, non-alcoholic steatohepatitis, morbid obesity

INTRODUCTION

Obesity is a disease that usually begins in childhood and it is becoming more frequent each day. It occurs as a result of an imbalance between calorie intake and energy expenditure. Obesity is defined by a body mass index (BMI) ≥ 30kg/m2 and morbid obesity as a BMI ≥ 40kg/m2. There are many factors involved in the development of obesity, including genetic and environmental factors. These factors can lead to the excessive accumulation of body fat and thereby to the onset of metabolic syndrome. Obesity reflects also a generalized proinflammatory state.

Recent research has shown that obesity, besides being a common risk factor for a wide range of diseases, including diabetes, cardiovascular disease and cancer, is associated with an increased risk of non-alcoholic fatty liver disease (NAFLD). Scientific evidence also demonstrates that obesity contributes to the progression of different types of liver diseases. Actually, it represents a risk factor for developing hepatocellular carcinoma (HCC) together with insulin resistance (IR). NAFLD is 6 times more frequent in obese patients than in normal population. Up to 75% of patients with obesity have some degree of fatty deposits in the liver, which can reach 100% when these patients present morbid obesity.

The prevalence of NAFLD has risen in the last decades, similarly to obesity and type 2 diabetes mellitus (T2D), becoming the most common chronic liver disease worldwide. NAFLD has a reported prevalence of 10 to 46% in Europe and in the United States, while the median prevalence reported worldwide is around 20%. The treatment of NAFLD is based on weight loss through lifestyle modifications, pharmacologic therapy and bariatric surgery. Bariatric surgery does not only contribute to weight loss, but it also improves the co-morbidities associated to obesity, such as T2D and pathological liver histological changes like hepatic inflammation and fibrosis.

DEFINITION OF NAFLD AND NASH

NAFLD is defined as an excessive fatty deposit in the hepatocytes in the absence of alcohol intake and of other known causes of fatty liver. NAFLD ranges from simple steatosis to non-alcoholic steatohepatitis (NASH) and even cirrhosis.

NAFL (non-alcoholic fatty liver) hepatic steatosis is present without evidence of significant inflammation, with > 5% of hepatocytes infiltrated with fat. This deposit of fat in the hepatic parenchyma is pathological when it exceeds 5% of the weight of the liver and other viral or metabolic liver diseases and the consumption of alcohol have been ruled out.

In **NASH** (non-alcoholic steatohepatitis) hepatic steatosis is associated with hepatic inflammation that may be histologically indistinguishable from alcoholic steatohepatitis. This condition will be determinant for the development of liver fibrosis and cancer.

Approximately 10 - 25% of patients with NAFLD will develop NASH, and 5 - 8% of those will develop liver cirrhosis within 5 years. After alcoholism and viral infections, NAFLD is the third main cause of liver cirrhosis.

ETIOLOGY

Hepatic steatosis is caused by the excessive accumulation of toxic lipids in the liver, including triglycerides, free fatty acids (FFA), ceramides and free cholesterol. This accumulation can result from the excessive importation of FFA from adipose tissue, from diminished hepatic export of FFA or from impaired beta-oxidation of FFA.

Although NAFLD has been considered the hepatic manifestation of the metabolic syndrome, new researches have shown that the association between NAFLD and metabolic syndrome is bidirectional. Insulin resistance (IR) and chronic inflammation are primarily responsible for these two entities.

The most important mechanisms in hepatic steatosis involve increased visceral adipose tissue, secretion of proinflammatory cytokines and adipokines and release of FFA into the portal system and systemic circulation, causing dyslipidemia and systemic IR. Therefore, IR, dyslipidemia and T2D could play a role in the etiopathogenesis of this entity. Given the importance of visceral adipose tissue, surveillance for patients with NAFLD should take into account an indicator of visceral obesity, and not only rely on BMI. Increases in visceral adipose tissue and intrahepatic fat correlate with increased gluconeogenesis, increased FFA levels and IR. Visceral fat is also associated with liver inflammation and fibrosis in patients with NASH, irrespective of IR, possibly through the mediation of interleukin-6 (a proinflammatory cytokine).

The main pathogenic factor related to steatosis is the increased flow and hepatic uptake of non-esterified fatty acids from excessive peripheral lipolysis, as a consequence of peripheral IR. Research has proved that adipose tissue (especially visceral adipose tissue) is subject to a state of chronic inflammation, with the ability to secrete adipokines. This fact has allowed to relate hepatic inflammation and the metabolic disorders that lead to the accumulation of triglycerides. NAFLD may also be present together with some endocrine diseases, such as polycystic ovary syndrome, hypothyroidism, growth hormone deficiency or hypercortisolism.

Clinical Features

NAFLD usually occurs between the fourth and sixth decade of life. Most patients are clinically asymptomatic, although some of them may complain of fatigue, dyspepsia, and vague right upper abdominal discomfort. Regarding physical findings, some patients may have hepatomegaly due to fatty infiltration of the liver, but this is not a common finding and it might be related to patients with more advanced disease. We could also find stigmata of chronic liver disease in patients who have developed cirrhosis.

DIAGNOSIS

The diagnosis of NAFLD requires to rule out any history of alcohol abuse (< 30g/day in men and < 20g/day in women) and other causes of hepatic steatosis, such as hepatitis C virus infection, autoimmune hepatitis, Wilson's disease, medication use, starvation, parenteral nutrition, etc.

Methods for diagnosing NAFLD can be divided into non-invasive and invasive. Among the non-invasive we find laboratory tests and radiographic examinations. As for invasive methods, we refer mainly to liver biopsy, which is the gold standard for the diagnosis of NAFLD. Furthermore liver biopsy is the only method available to differentiate NAFL from NASH.

Most patients with NAFL or mild NASH are asymptomatic and NAFLD is detected accidentally in a routine analysis. Actually elevated liver enzymes are detected in approximately 20% of NAFLD patients.

Regarding **laboratory tests,** aspartate aminotransferase (AST) and alanine aminotransferase (ALT) levels can be normal or moderately elevated. Also an AST: ALT ratio < 1 supports the diagnosis of NASH. Besides liver enzymes, the following tests should also be obtained: anti-hepatitis C virus antibody, hepatitis A IgG, hepatitis B surface antigen, surface antibody and core antibody. We should also obtain iron levels, ferritin, and total iron binding capacity. Finally there is a series of parameters related to autoimmune hepatitis that should be assessed, such as serum gammaglobulin level or antinuclear body. However laboratory tests might be normal, and when they show any abnormality, they are not sufficient for making the diagnosis. In terms of **radiographic examinations,** ultrasound is the most available method and it represents the first-line diagnostic tool for detecting liver steatosis. It is a useful tool for diagnosing moderate to severe degree hepatic steatosis, but its accuracy is limited regarding mild steatosis. There are other methods that are also used, such as computed tomography (CT), magnetic resonance (MRI) and proton magnetic resonance spectroscopy (MRS). CT has limitations such as the fact that there is a potential risk related to its radiation and it has also a limited accuracy in detecting mild steatosis. MRI and MRS provide a highly accurate and reproducible diagnosis for evaluating NAFLD.

We must also take into account FibroScan, which is used to assess liver fibrosis by measuring liver stiffness.

Nevertheless, as non-invasive methods cannot make a distinction between simple steatosis and NASH, liver biopsy remains necessary, especially when radiographic examinations are not consistent with fatty infiltration, when other causes for steatosis have not been excluded or when the patient has signs or symptoms of cirrhosis.

As for **liver biopsy**, it remains the gold standard for the diagnosis of NAFLD and it represents the only method to confirm the diagnosis of NASH as well as for establishing the different stages of fibrosis. However it is only performed when the diagnosis remains unclear after obtaining laboratory tests and hepatic imaging, or if the information provided by the biopsy might condition the patient's treatment. The reason why this technique is so restrictively indicated is that it constitutes an invasive method with possible serious complications. In addition, histological alterations of the liver are not distributed homogeneously and the biopsy may be unrepresentative.

TREATMENT

Although the optimal treatment has yet to be elucidated, the treatment of NAFLD is focused on weight loss. For achieving this goal we count on three therapeutic weapons that can be complementary: lifestyle modifications, pharmacologic therapy and bariatric surgery. The main goal of these therapies is to slow down or stop the disease progression, whether it is in its earliest stages or in the stage of fibrosis or cirrhosis.

For the inflammatory parameters of the liver to improve, patients must lose at least 5% of their total weight. If weight loss exceeds 7%, NASH may be resolved. However, to reduce the degree of liver fibrosis, patients must lose at least 10% of their total weight.

The improvement of NAFLD is directly proportional to the weight loss, regardless of whether it has been achieved through lifestyle changes or bariatric surgery.

Lifestyle Modification

First line therapy for NAFLD includes lifestyle changes aimed at weight loss through low-calorie diets and physical exercise. Weight loss leads to a reduction in both visceral adipose tissue and IR. There are different publications that show a significant reduction of hepatic steatosis after the implantation of lifestyle changes, as well as an improvement in IR and BMI.

It is not clear what kind of exercise is the most beneficial, but it has been shown that adding physical exercise to a low-calorie diet can enhance the benefits in the management of NAFLD and IR, regardless of weight loss.

Pharmacologic Therapy

Nowadays there is not any drug specifically accepted for the treatment of NAFLD, with weight loss being the only treatment that has proved to be effective.

Metformin has beneficial effects in preventing diabetes onset and leads to mild weight loss. These two effects are also beneficial for NAFLD patients, although metformin has not proved to have a direct effect on liver histology.

Another pharmacologic option would be pioglitazone, which also helps in improving IR and histological hepatic disease activity. However, due to its side effects, its general application is not recommended.

Bariatric Surgery

In Europe and North America, the prevalence of NAFLD among patients whose BMI overcomes 40Kg/m2 ranges between 75% an 100%. However, NAFLD alone does not constitute an indication for bariatric surgery at the moment.

Weight loss, regardless the way it is achieved, is the most important factor related to the improvement in the histological characteristics of patients with NAFLD. In fact, this improvement is directly proportional to the weight lost. In this regard, bariatric surgery allows the patient to achieve a greater and sustained weight loss over time. In addition, the main etiologic factors involved in the development of NAFLD are obesity and IR, and there is scientific evidence that bariatric surgery is effective both for weight loss and for the resolution of diabetes mellitus type 2.

As for the most recommended bariatric surgery technique, sleeve gastrectomy and gastrointestinal bypass techniques have proved to be superior to gastric banding in terms of weight loss.

It is important to take into account the stage of liver disease in obese patients with NAFLD undergoing bariatric surgery, since liver cirrhosis is associated with increased postoperative morbidity and mortality. Furthermore it is also important to bear in mind that the mortality of these patients decreases as the experience of both the medical and surgical team increases.

In the case of obese patients with NAFLD presenting Child-Pugh class A liver cirrhosis without portal hypertension or decompensation, both sleeve gastrectomy and gastrointestinal bypass are recommended. However, it should be borne in mind that some publications describe that gastrointestinal bypass techniques can lead to the massive destruction of adipocytes and an important increase in the levels of free fatty acids that are taken up by the liver, which results in worsening of steatosis, steatohepatitis, or even cirrhosis.

Fortunately this complication was rather related to more aggressive techniques that are no longer performed as the jejunoileal bypass procedure, and it is exceptional to find it after the completion of a Roux-en-Y gastric bypass (RYGB), which is the most common derivative technique today. Nevertheless, since sleeve gastrectomy (SG) does not have a derivative component, it is considered to be more physiological and has less risk of hepatic decompensation both during the immediate postoperative period and during the weight loss that takes place after surgery.

It also allows endoscopic access to the gastric sleeve and duodenum, which may be important depending on the evolution of the hepatopathy of these patients.

Therefore, in obese patients who have developed cirrhosis, surgical treatment will be conditioned by the stage of liver disease presented by the patient, which will be measured using the Child-Pugh scale or the MELD-Score. We must bear in mind that patients with decompensated cirrhosis should not undergo bariatric surgery given the high risk of potentially serious and even fatal complications.

Bariatric surgery using mixed procedures (restrictive and malabsorptive) as a Roux-en-Y gastric bypass, improves liver abnormalities associated with non alcoholic fatty liver disease in morbidly obese patients.

Kalinowski et al. studied the evolution of NAFLD and NASH using intraoperative liver biopsies in patients who underwent bariatric surgery (SG vs RYGB). Patients who underwent SG showed significant improvements in AST, ALT, and gamma-glutamyltransferase at 12 months which revealed a greater improvement in liver abnormalities and inflammation for SG.

Praveen Raj and coworkers showed a greater improvement of steatosis, lobular inflammation, ballooning degeneration and fibrosis among patients with NAFLD who underwent a sleeve gastrectomy in comparison to a Roux-en-Y gastric bypass.

CONCLUSION

We can conclude that it is important to analyze through further studies the benefit of bariatric surgery in patients with NAFLD and high risk of developing cirrhosis, given the existing evidence that these techniques improve both liver steatosis and fibrosis, besides contributing to weight loss and the improvement of insulin resistance.

REFERENCES

Aller, R. Consensus document. Management of Non-alcoholic fatty liver disease: Clinical guidelines. *Gastroenterol. Hepatol.,* 2018;41(5):328 - 349.

Brunner, K. T., Henneberg, C. J., Wilechansky, R. M. et al. Nonalcoholic Fatty Liver Disease and Obesity Treatment. *Curr. Obes. Rep.,* 2019 Apr. 3. doi: 10.1007/s13679-019-00345-1.

Brunt, E. M., Tiniakos, D. G. Alcoholic and non-alcoholic fatty liver disease. In: Surgical pathology of the GI tract, liver, biliary tract and pancreas, 2nd ed. Odze, R. D., Goldblum, J. R. (Eds), Elsevier, Philadelphia 2009. P. 1007.

Buqué, X., Aspichueta, P., Ochoa, B. Molecular basis of obesity-related liver steatosis. *Rev. Esp. Enferm. Dig.,* 2008; 100: 565 - 578.

Caldwell, S. H., Oelsner, D. H., Iezzoni, J. C. et al. Cryptogenic cirrhosis: clinical characterization and risk factors for underlying disease. *Hepatology,* 1999; 29:664.

Chalasani, N., Younossi, Z., Lavine, J. E. et al. The diagnosis and management of nonalcoholic fatty liver disease: Practice guidance from the American Association for the Study of Liver diseases. *Hepatology,* 2018; 67:328.

Dietrich, P., Hellerbrand, C. Non-alcoholic fatty liver disease, obesity and the metabolic syndrome. *Best Practice and Research Clinical Gastroenterology,* 2014; 28:637 - 653.

Donnelly, K. L., Smith, C. I., Schwarzenberg, S. J. et al. Sources of fatty acids stored in iver and secreted via lipoproteins in patients with non-alcoholic fatty liver disease. *J. Clin. Invest.,* 2005; 115:1343.

European Association for the Study of the Liver (EASL), European Association for the Study of Diabetes (EASD), European Association for the Study of Obesity (EASO). EASL-EASD-EASO Clinical Practice

Guidelines for the management of non-alcoholic fatty liver disease. *J. Hepatol.,* 2016; 64:1388.

Graffy, P. M., Pickhardt, P. J. Quantification of hepatic and visceral fat by CT and MR imaging: relevance to the obesity epidemic, metabolic syndrome and NAFLD. *Br. J. Radiol.,* 2016; 89: 20151024.

Hannah, W. N., Jr., Harrison, S. A. Effect of Weight Loss, Diet, Exercise, and Bariatric Surgery on Nonalcoholic Fatty Liver Disease. *Clinics in liver disease,* 2016;20(2):339 - 350.

Ipsen, D. H., Lykkesfeldt, J., Tveden-Nyborg, P. Molecular mechanisms of hepatic lipid accumulation in non-alcoholic fatty liver disease. *Cellular and Molecular Life Sciences,* 2018; 75: 3313 - 3327.

Jan, A., Narwaria, M., Mahawar, K. K. A Systematic Review of Bariatric Surgery in Patients with Liver Cirrhosis. *Obes. Surg.,* 2015; 25(8): 1518 - 1526.

Kalinowski, P., Paluszkiewicz, R., Wróblewski, T. et al. Ghrelin, leptin, and glycemic control after sleeve gastrectomy versus Roux-en-Y gastric bypass—results of a randomized clinical trial. *Surg. Obes. Relat. Dis.,* 2017; 13:181 - 188.

Kneeman, J. M., Misdraji, J., Corey, K. E. Secondary causes of nonalcoholic fatty liver disease. *Therap. Adv. Gastroenterol.,* 2012; 5(3):199 - 207.

Lee, H. W., Kim, K. J., Jung, K. S. et al. The relationship between visceral obesity and hepatic steatosis measured by controlled attenuation parameter. *PloS ONE*, 2017; 12 (10): e0187066.

Lee, D. H. Imaging evaluation of non-alcoholic fatty liver disease: focused on quantification. *Clin. Mol. Hepatol.,* 2017; 23: 290 - 301.

Ludwig, J., Viggiano, T. R., McGill, D. B. et al. Nonalcoholic steatohepatitis: Mayo Clinic experiences with a hitherto unnamed disease. *Mayo Clin. Proc.,* 1980; 55:434.

Marino, L., Jornayvaz, F. R. Endocrine causes of nonalcoholic fatty liver disease. *World J. Gastroenterol.,* 2015; 21(39):11053 - 11076.

Matteoni, C. A., Younossi, Z. M., Gramlich, T. et al. Nonalcoholic fatty liver disease: a spectrum of clinical and pathological severity. *Gastroenterology,* 1999; 116:1413.

Milic, S., Lulic, D., Stimac, D. Non-alcoholic fatty liver disease and obesity: Biochemical, metabolic and clinical presentations. *World J. Gastroenterol.,* 2014; 20 (28): 9330 - 9337.

Miquilena Colina, M. E., García Monzón, C. Obesity and fatty liver. *Gastroenterol. Hepatol.,* 2011;10:5.

Miquilena Colina, M. E., García Monzón, C. Obesity and liver disease. *Gastroenterol. Hepatol.,* 2010:33:591 - 604.

Nassir, F., Rector, R. S., Hammoud, G. M. et al. Pathogenesis and Prevention of Hepatic Steatosis. *Gastroenterology and Hepatology,* 2015; 11: 167 - 175.

Neuschwander Tetri, B. A., Caldwell, S. H. Nonalcoholic steatohepatitis: summary of an AASLD Single Topic Conference. *Hepatology,* 2003; 37:1202.

Praveen, Raj P., Gomes, R. M., Kumar, S. et al. The effect of surgically induced weight loss on nonalcoholic fatty liver disease in morbidly obese Indians: "NASHOST" prospective observational trial. *Surg. Obes. Relat. Dis.,* 2015; 11(6): 1315 - 22.

Promrat, K., Kleiner, D. E., Niemeier, H. M. et al. Randomized Controlled Trial Testing the Effects of Weight Loss on Nonalcoholic Steatohepatitis (NASH). *Hepatology,* (Baltimore, Md). 2010; 51(1):121 - 129.

Sanders, F. W. B., Acharjee, A., Walker, C., et al. Hepatic steatosis risk is partly driven by increased de novo lipogenesis following carbohydrate consumption. *Genome Biology*, (2018) 19:79.

Sheth, S. G., Gordon, F. D., Chopra, S. Nonalcoholic steatohepatitis. *Ann. Intern. Med.,* 1997; 126:137.

Van der Poorten, D., Milner, K. L., Hui, J. et al. Visceral fat: a key mediator of steatohepatitis in metabolic liver disease. *Hepatology,* 2008; 48:449.

Vargas, V., Allende, H., Lecube, A. et al. Surgically induced weight loss by gastric bypass improves non alcoholic fatty liver disease in morbid obese patients. *World J. Hepatol.,* 2012; 4(12):382 -8.

Vilar-Gomez, E., Martinez-Perez, Y., Calzadilla-Bertot, L. et al. Weight Loss Through Lifestyle Modification Significantly Reduces Features of Nonalcoholic Steatohepatitis. *Gastroenterology,* 2015; 149(2):367 - 378.

In: Liver Steatosis and Bariatric Surgery ISBN: 978-1-53616-444-2
Editors: Jaime Ruiz-Tovar et al.

Chapter 3

FATTY LIVER DEVELOPMENT: IMBALANCE BETWEEN ACQUISITION AND REMOVAL OF LIPIDS

Lorea Zubiaga*[*], *MD, PhD
Lille University, Inserm-U1190, EGID, CHU Lille. Lille, France

ABSTRACT

Fatty liver, hepatic steatosis and Nonalcoholic fatty liver disease (NAFLD) is an umbrella of terms used to describe a range of related disorders characterized by the deposition of triglycerides as droplets in the cytoplasm of hepatocytes. The fatty liver is now considered a multifaceted complex systemic condition. Moreover, recent evidence suggests that this steatosis may progress to an advanced liver fibrosis challenging the previous dogma that "*steatosis is a benign condition*". High levels of insulin and insulin resistance are often associated with hepatic steatosis and although it is necessary, is not sufficient for the disease debut and progress. NAFLD, obesity, Type 2 Diabetes and Metabolic syndrome are linked by a vicious circle which induce several difficulties in the metabolic control and where bariatric and metabolic surgery has changed many paradigms.

[*] Corresponding Author's Email: loreazubiaga@gmail.com.

Keywords: fatty liver, western diet, *de novo* lipogenesis, fatty acids, very low density lipoprotein, insulin resistance

INTRODUCTION

Fatty liver is the most frequent chronic hepatic disease in developed countries and its prevalence runs in parallels the rise in obesity, type 2 diabetes (T2D) and metabolic syndrome (MetS). This disease is associated to the modern life and its most common interpretation is related to over-nutrition and consumption of well-known western diet [1]. However, the fatty liver can also be induced by endocrine disorders, viral infections or side effects of pharmacological therapies. In most cases it is an ailment that causes no symptoms and it moves silently generating tissue damage to liver parenchyma, which can lead to fibrosis as NASH, them cirrhosis and finally the liver failure [2].

Fatty liver begins with the aberrant accumulation of triglycerides (TG) in the liver. The pathogenesis of this disease remains poorly understood and its evolution of the liver steatosis is directly interconnected to classic components of the metabolic syndrome as: hyperglycemia, hyper-insulinemia, insulin resistance and hypertriglyceridemia [3]. However, most of the patients with fatty liver display all of these conditions independent of body weight [4]. In fact, the "lean NAFLD" phenotype has a renewed interest among researchers. This fact is due to that this condition developments selectively increase in visceral adiposity without changes in the body mass index and, sometimes, even with normal waist circumference [5]. This "lean NAFLD" patient develops metabolic problems and cardiovascular disease similarly to obese patients and this is a worrisome problem, because these patients are difficult to diagnose and even more difficult to treat [6]. However, the "lean NAFLD" allow us to study the genetic component of this disease. A recent publication confirms that the fatty liver development and progression derive from a complex interplay between genetic and environmental factor [7], and we should probably distinguish a strong genetic component of the disease from the metabolic origin as such as in the diabetes (type 1 diabetes/MODY/T2D) [8]. However, in this assessment we will focus on the physiopathology hypotheses of this disease that are closer to obesity, concentrating the concepts on the damage associated with environmental rather than genetic causes and without entering the complex world of inflammatory and immunological signals that also accompany this disease.

Assumptions and Data

Fatty Acids as a Regular Fuel for Energy

As a central regulator of lipid homeostasis, the liver is responsible for directing the synthesis of new fatty acids, their export and subsequent redistribution to other tissues, as well as their utilization as energy substrates [9]. Nearly all forms of fatty acids have an even number of carbon atoms and they can be presented as individual fatty acids or free fatty acids (FFA) and also as non-esterified fatty acids (NEFA) [10]. Fatty acids are the foremost metabolic fuel in the body and they play a central role providing energy to the majority of tissues (except brain, which use glucose) particularly during fasting.

Circulating FFA are reabsorbed in various organs where, if not oxidized, they accumulate as intra-cytoplasmic droplets of TG or like some lipid intermediates, such as the diacyl-glycerols (DAG), molecules which, sometimes can promote cell lipotoxicity [11]. In the liver, the major storage form of FFA is in triglycerides (TG) shape. The selection of TG as energy resource in the body comes from two physicochemical properties: TG provides greater caloric density (9 kcal/g) than other substrates (4 kcal/g from carbohydrates or proteins) and they can accumulate to high levels in the cell with no adverse osmotic or colloidal effects. However, the lipids accumulation on the liver is defined as the deposition of TG as droplets in the cytoplasm of hepatocytes in more that 5% of these cells [12].

Buildup of Lipids in the Liver Is a Normal Response to Fasting

Hepatic lipid accumulation occurs transiently as a metabolic adaptation to continuous food deprivation (fasting or starvation). In humans, this period normally corresponds to 12–24 h without food intake [13]. In the first phase of fasting, the hepatic glucose output is derived both from gluconeogenesis and glycogenolysis. Both process entail a reduction of glycogen stores in the liver. However, if an extra demand of energy occurs during this period, hormonal signals stimulate adipose tissue to release NEFA into circulation to address to the liver where they will be used as energy substrates. Within a prolonged period of fasting the reduction of hepatic glycogen stores further stimulates adipose tissue lipolysis. This feedback is essential to maintain a constant supply of energy to the body [9]. During this process the liver upregulates expression of the hepatic fatty acid transporter. Fatty acids in the liver act as main substrate for the oxidative process and to generate ketones. In this way, the liver maintains two mechanisms that prevent the oxidation of amino acids in the hepatic parenchyma. Avoiding oxidation of amino acids is essential for normal functions in the cells. During a period of starvation (fasting periods prolonged for more than 60 hours) the accumulation of hepatic lipids is higher but also begins the second phase of the liver as an energy provider through the transformation of those lipids into molecules that can travel to other organs and make up for the energy deficit (as ketone bodies and lipoproteins) [14]. In this sense, the lipid stockpiling in the liver and the transformation of them in energy seems to be a protective mechanism to all body when food intake is compromised [13].

The mechanisms that promote the liver fat piling up are not fully elucidated but it has been hypothesized that when the fatty acids acquisitions exceeds the capacity for removal them, these fatty acids are over-stored. The fatty acids used for hepatic TG formation are derived from three sources: (1) diet, (2) De Novo synthesis, and from (3) the adipose tissue. In the other side, fatty acids that arrives to the liver parenchyma have three major destinations: (a) They can be oxidized to produce energy and ketone bodies, (b) re-esterified to TG and stored in droplets, or (c) coupled to apolipoproteins and secreted as very-low-density lipoproteins (VLDL) [15]. An overview of each of these processes is described in Figure 1 and will be described below.

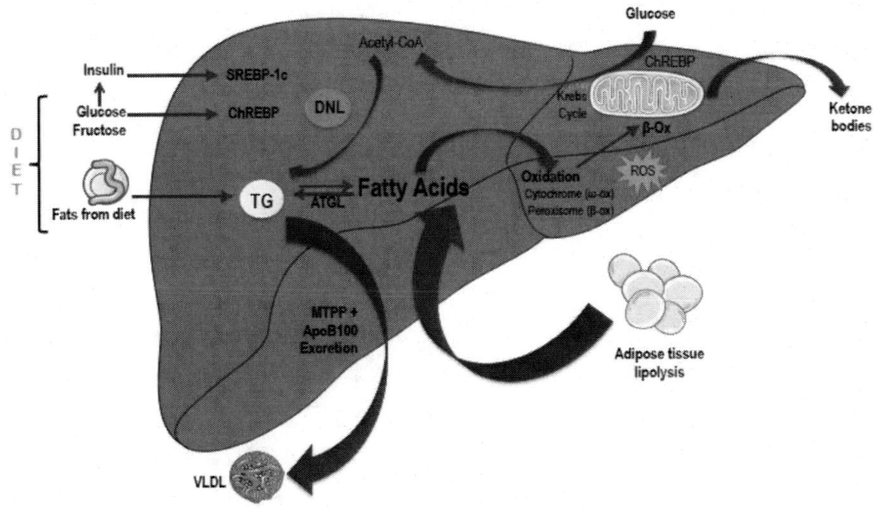

Figure 1. Lipid metabolism in the liver.. Processes that increase the entry of fatty acids and triglycerides or reduce their exit can cause hepatic steatosis. The main sources of FFA are: diet, endogenous synthesis and lipolysis in peripheral tissues. Carbohydrate intake increases glucose and insulin levels, which activate two transcription factors (ChREBP and SREBP-1c) in the liver that promote de novo lipogenesis (DNL). FFAs have several possible destinations within the hepatic parenchyma: 1) Esterified by adipose triglyceride lipase (ATGL) and stored as triglycerides (TG) in lipid droplets. 2) Metabolized by oxidation processes (B-ox or W-ox) forming substrates for a new synthesis (Acetyl-CoA) and also as reactive oxygen species (ROS). They can also form ketone bodies that are expelled into the circulation. 3) Packed with apoB100 by means of Microsomal triglyceride transfer protein (MTTP) and segregated in the blood as low-density lipoproteins (VLDL).

Fatty Liver and Diet

The increasing prevalence of fatty liver the increased in the general population over the past 40 years is due to changes in the quantity and composition of food. Specifically, has been attributed to the widespread availability of the so-called western diet that is rich in saturated fats and refined sugars [16]. The western diet (WD) is mainly described as a high-fat/high-sugar diet or specifically as high-cholesterol/sucrose (fructose) diet. Regardless of the combination of the elements that define the WD, what is relevant in this nutritional form is the fact that this diet promotes hepatic steatosis in conjunction with altered liver transcriptomic and metabolomic profiles. These altered profiles completely modify the signals that control liver functions, inducing phenomena that can be paradoxical. For example, giving the order to increase the internal storages when in reality there is already an excess of fats [1].

Analyzing in detail the effect of the WD it has described the influence of hypercaloric diets on fatty liver. Indeed, when talking about high-calorie diets, it is easy to understand diets rich in saturated fatty acids (SFA). However, the studies analyzing the hypercaloric point of view usually have been undertaken using different degrees of energy excess and the macronutrient of interest are the carbohydrates [2]. In fact, some of these studies have demonstrated that an acute consumption of a high-fructose diet leads to a significant increase in liver fat content [17]. The most plausible hypothesis for this phenomenon is that fructose consumption routes dietary carbons directly to the liver in a promptly manner to enter biosynthetic pathways, including De Novo lipogenesis (DNL) [18]. The way in which this process predisposes to fat accumulation will be described later in the reading. Nonetheless, when comparing hypercaloric diets enriched in either fructose or glucose it would appear that both influence liver fat accumulation in a similar manner [19]. The majority of carbohydrates in the WD coming from added extrinsic sugars (Ex. sucrose and corn syrup). The added sugars universally present in modern food are added to enhance the taste in some beverages and processed food and they are consumed unnoticed manner. Both sucrose and corn syrup are composed of approximately 50/50 proportion of fructose/glucose and these two sugars consumed in combination are more deleterious and more inclined to stimulates DNL than when they are taken isolated [20].

On the other hand, faced with the same amount of calories, the predominant effect is the composition of macronutrients in the diet. Thus, a diet composed mainly of SFA will be more harmful even if it has a lower calorie intake [2]. Diets rich in SFA cause an increase in the accumulation of hepatic TG, while diets rich in monounsaturated fatty acids (MUFA) or polyunsaturated fatty acids (PUFA) tend to decrease the TG in the liver. The mechanism by which the SFA lead to an accumulation of TG is not yet clarified, although it has been suggested that the lipotoxity of this kind of fat alters per se the oxidative stress of the cell (at the endoplasmic reticulum level and/or mitochondrial) [21]. There are also hypotheses that point to a disordered metabolism of phospholipids [22] or to alterations in the regulation of lipogenic genes, which promote the production and accumulation of TG. In general, all of these ideas pose a disturbance of liver to handle a high flow of lipids from the diets. As these lipids cannot enter the oxidation or lipoprotein production pathways, they accumulate in the parenchyma [11]. Supporting this idea, Koopman et al. reported that the accumulation of fat in the liver was noticeably greater when the same amount of calories were consumed in a greater number of intakes during the day; i.e., isocaloric high fat diets taken 5 times a day (meals + snacks) were more harmful than taken 3 times (meals) a day [23]. Therefore, in the development of fatty liver not only the number of calories is important, but also how they are distributed in relation to the composition of macronutrients, as well as the frequency with which these calories are ingested during the day.

Adipose Tissue Lipolysis and Hepatic Lipid Uptake

When energy demand exceeds metabolic energy from diet, NEFAs are mobilized from white adipose tissue (WAT) by the lipolysis. Lipolysis process is stimulated by the catecholamines while the insulin is the key signal to inhibit it. During fasting and intense exercise, insulin levels are low, allowing norepinephrine, cortisol and growth hormone to synergistically stimulate lipolysis from the WAT, allowing an increase of circulating fatty acid availability [24]. Hormonally regulated lipolysis depends on the activity of the lipolytic enzyme, hormone-sensitive lipase (HSL). Insulin and catecholamines from sympathetic nervous system (SNS) modulate HSL activity by decreasing and increasing respectively the energetic signals coming from the adipocytes. SNS activity also stimulates cortisol release. The metabolic response of WAT to corticoids also depends on the duration of exposure, where chronic stimulation induces the lipolysis by transcriptionally regulation of HSL [25]. Excessive lipolysis and adipose tissue fatty acid release into circulation results in ectopic accumulation of lipids as liver and the vascular system.

In obesity, as in fasting periods, there is a rise in sympathetic activity and adipose tissue lipolysis [26]. This increased lipolytic response is associated to the excess of the adiposity, characterized by a decreased lipolytic capacity in subcutaneous adipose tissue and an increased lipolysis from VAT [27]. In subcutaneous adipose tissue, obesity decreases HSL expression, limiting sensitivity to adrenergic stimulation. However, in obesity there is an increase of sensitivity to catecholamine-induced lipolysis in the visceral fat so, catecholamine-stimulated lipolysis depends on the regional adipose tissue depot. The reduction of the lipolytic hormone expression along with increased adipose tissue mass results in more adipose-tissue-derived fatty acids entering circulation in obese than in normal-weight individuals [28]. Moreover, in obesity the clearance by skeletal muscle is decreased. This phenomenon allows the increased lipolysis in the adipose tissue results in hyperlipidemia and an increased hepatic lipid uptake, which, is critical for the development of hepatic TG accumulation [29].

De novo Lipogenesis

Hepatic *De novo* lipogenesis (DNL) is the biochemical process of fatty acids synthesis from acetyl-CoA subunits coming from different pathways, most commonly from glycolysis and carbohydrate catabolism [30]. The DNL is driven by two transcription factors that are widely expressed in the liver and in the adipose tissue: the Sterol Response Element Binding Protein 1c (SREBP1c) and the Carbohydrate Response Element Binding Protein (ChREBP). Both factors regulate expression of key lipogenic genes to produce the fatty-acid synthase and the acetyl-CoA carboxylase, the two key enzymes of DNL. These enzymes use the acetyl-CoA and the malonyl-CoA derived from glucose catabolism (or other carbon precursors) to generate palmitate [31]. Usually, the palmitate has detrimental effects in the body; however, the palmitate synthesized by DNL, can be modified by endogenous enzymes to produce multiple lipid species that are easily to storage [32].

Under normal physiological conditions, an increase of circulating glucose is followed by a rise in lipogenic enzyme expression, which stimulates hepatic glucose clearance and storage of the carbons as fatty acids and TG. Carbohydrates in general and specially glucose regulate directly the ChREBP activity. In the same sense, postprandial hyperglycemia leads to increase circulating insulin and this hormone stimulates SREBP1c in the liver. Thus, the hyperglycemic and hyperinsulinemic conditions are closely linked to DLN. In addition, SREBP1c indirectly contributes to the development of hepatic insulin resistance, since enhanced lipogenesis and subsequent accumulation of harmful lipid species, such as DAG, which in turn may interfere with insulin signaling [11].

While glucose is the main substrate for DNL, fructose is a highly lipogenic substrate which can provides an extended number of carbons. The importance of fructose as a lipogenic substrate comes from the main function of the liver in fructose clearance. In the first pass of portal circulation after meal ingestion, the liver sequesters 71% of dietary fructose, while only takes 13% of glucose [33]. Moreover, fructose is phosphorylated at carbon 1 rather than carbon 6, so it cannot be used to synthesize glycogen but instead is quantitatively converted to glyceraldehyde-3-phosphate, providing the main substrate for DLN. Similarly, fructose may bypass the critical regulatory step catalyzed by phosphofructokinase-1 in glycolysis [34] so it can enter directly to biosynthesis reactions. Even more, fructose also potentiates glucose-stimulated insulin secretion and also increases the activation of ChREBP. In this way, a diet rich in fructose increases ChREBP binding to DNA nearly four fold [35]. This has implications that mean fructose may reinforce some of the pathogenic mechanisms leading to fatty liver via DLN.

Another pathway associated with DLN is mediated by excess in glucocorticoids. The 11β-hydroxysteroid dehydrogenase type 1 (11β-HSD1) is a key enzyme that catalyzes the intracellular conversion of cortisone to physiologically active cortisol and it is an NADPH-dependent enzyme highly expressed in key metabolic tissues as the liver and the adipose tissue. The expression of this enzyme is up-regulated in obesity leading to an excess of glucocorticoid production cortisol overproduction from adipose tissue is an important stimulus for the liver's lipogenic pathways, however local liver cortisol production is much more active to stimulate the fatty acids production. In fat, corticoids contribute to driving hepatic steatosis by decreasing lipid oxidation and increasing DNL and TG esterification [13].

Fatty Acids Oxidation and Ketogenesis

Oxidation of fatty acids occurs principally in the mitochondria, providing a source of energy to generate ATP especially when circulating glucose levels are low. During this process, fatty acid chains are broken apart into acetic acid fragments and generates acetyl-CoA molecules that are further oxidized by the citric acid cycle (TCA/Krebs cycle) to produce carbon dioxide and water and release energy. This process is traditionally called Beta-oxidation (β-ox). β-ox is primarily facilitated by the hepatocytes mitochondria due the action of the mitochondrial tri-functional protein (MTP), an enzyme that catalyzes the last 3 steps of this process [36]. Hepatic β-ox in response to lipid accumulation prevents lipotoxicity and providing extra energy when in periods of starvation, the gluconeogenesis is insufficient. In this sense, limiting β-ox process is usually associated to a severe exacerbation of hepatic lipid accumulation [37].

However, the oxidation also can be developed in the cytoplasm by the peroxisomes (β-ox) or cytochromes (ω-ox). These two last settings usually are activated due to mitochondria lack the ability to oxidize very long chain fatty acids or when exists environments with lipid overload. However, these two processes generate considerable amounts of reactive oxygen species (ROS), oxidative stress, and toxic dicarboxylic acids, potentially promoting inflammation and hepatic damage [15]. Indeed, lipid oxidation by these pathways can produce a damage into mitochondrial DNA further diminish mitochondrial function, establishing a self-perpetuating vicious cycle to exacerbate mitochondrial dysfunction and oxidative stress [38].

DNL is usually responsible for the steatosis resulting from high-frutose diets. However, fructose can also promotes the inhibition of β-ox via carnitine palmitoyltransferase I (CPT1) activity inhibition. This enzyme regulates the formation of acyl-carnitines by catalyzing the transfer of the acyl group of a long-chain fatty acyl-CoA from coenzyme A to l-carnitine. The resulting product is often Palmitoylcarnitine the first committed intermediate produced during fatty acid synthesis. But, inhibition of CPT1 resulting increases malonyl-CoA synthesis and chronically downregulates the expression of beta-oxidative genes [13]. One again, the hepatic lipid accumulation resulting from dietary fructose also affects another process, which is key in the lipids distribution.

β-ox is upregulated in the post-absorptive state and reduced in the postprandial state, a response mediated by systemic substrate and hormone concentrations. For example, the glucagon stimulates β-ox by upregulation of peroxisome proliferator-activated receptor α (PPARα) activity, while insulin and glucose downregulates β-ox by suppressing adipose tissue TG lipolysis, reducing the delivery of fatty acids to the liver and increasing hepatic DNL [11]. Thus, obesity can causes a decrease in beta-oxidation, which contributes to lipid accumulation [38].

Ketogenesis is the catabolic process for ketone bodies production through breakdown of fatty acids. This process supplies energy under circumstances such as fasting or caloric restriction to certain organs, particularly the brain, heart and skeletal muscle. This event is notably important when the gluconeogenesis process is insufficient and can cause hypoglycemia. As energy requirements are urgent the liver oxidizes fats and manufactures ketone bodies [39]. Ketogenesis occurs constantly in a compensatory amount in healthy individuals but it can also take place when there is insufficient insulin (Ex. in type 1 diabetes), particularly during periods of "ketogenic stress". In these cases, pushing the body to chronically supply itself with energy from ketone bodies can create a lethal condition called ketoacidosis. Fatty acids are enzymatically broken down in β-ox to form acetyl-CoA. However, if the amounts of acetyl-CoA generated in this process overwhelm the capacity of the TCA cycle, acetyl-CoA is then used instead in biosynthesis of ketone bodies. Hepatic ketogenesis could potentially contribute to control and avoid fatty liver pathogenesis, because it is activated in states of FFA circulation and diminished carbohydrate availability concentrations are very low. But, in obesity the raised FFA levels exceed the ketogenic machinery as various substrates and enzymes from this process cannot be recycled at the same rate as they are consumed. On the other hand, hyperglycemia acts as inhibitor of ketogenesis. In both pathways, the decrease of ketone bodies production rate allows the lipids accumulation in the liver [37].

Liver Lipoprotein Management

A central metabolic role of the liver is to maintain plasma glucose within narrow physiological limits regardless of the nutritional state of the animal. In energy excess, glucose is converted to fatty acids, which are further used to synthesize TG. Hepatic TG derives from: 1) uptake of circulating fatty acids; 2) uptake of circulating remnants of VLDL and chylomicron (lipase action); and 3) through the hepatic DNL TG can be stored or incorporated into very-low-density lipoproteins (VLDL) and secreted into the blood. VLDL synthesis by the liver involves complex processes such as synthesis and the coordinated assembly of protein components (apolipoproteins) and of hydrophilic (phospholipids, free cholesterol) and hydrophobic (triacylglycerols (TAG), cholesteryl esters) lipid components. VLDL particles are formed in the endoplasmic reticulum, where apolipoprotein B100 (apoB100) is lipidated in a process catalyzed by the enzyme microsomal triglyceride transfer protein (MTTP) [40]. Consequently, apoB100 and MTTP are key elements in hepatic VLDL secretion and in maintaining hepatic lipid homeostasis and some genetic defect in one of these 2 elements is associated with the presence of fatty liver. The production and transport of the VLDL is an efficient source of energy either for storage in adipose tissue or for its utilization by muscles [41].

The precise mechanisms responsible for the close relationship between fatty liver and obesity are still unknown, but is evident to think that if exist a blockade of hepatic VLDL production and secretion, this situation results in an accumulation of TG in the liver favoring the development of fatty liver. However, other hypotheses have been proposed with the insulin in the target. Postprandial insulin can suppress hepatic VLDL production by a number of mechanisms, including the down-regulation of the MTTP gene expression, increasing degradation of apoB within hepatocytes and inhibiting the maturation of VLDL. However, the suppressive effect of insulin on VLDL production is reversed in chronic hyperinsulinemia conditions. In addition, it has been reported that high levels of insulin plus insulin-resistence do not decrease the production of the VLDL, but instead they stimulated it [42] as in obesity, T2D and MetS. In this sense, the IR of adipose tissue leads to higher circulating NEFA concentrations, and an increased FFA flux to the liver stimulating hepatic TG synthesis so, lipids storages increase in a first stage of fatty liver. The excess of lipids in the liver parenchyma also impairs hepatic extraction of insulin. Hepatic insulin resistance is also linked to an increasing TG synthesis and VLDL production and secretion as VLDL-TG. Despite higher VLDL-TG secretion in patients with fatty liver, regular VLDL-apoB100 secretion did not change, suggesting that hepatic steatosis patients do not secrete additional, but instead larger and more TG-rich, VLDL particles. Nevertheless, enormous VLDL particles cannot be secreted when they have a diameter that exceeds that of the sinusoidal endothelial pores [11]. This situation can be another cause for lipids accumulation in the liver parenchyma.

Glucoregulatory Hormones

Insulin

Most patients with fatty liver have hyperinsulinemia and IR at the same time, leaving to glimpse that insulin seems to be associated in several disturbances in the called metabolic diseases [43]. In fact, postprandial hyperinsulinemia is present in 100% of NAFLD individuals and usually is independent of diabetes status [44]. Insulin promotes the DLN and glycerol-neogenesis, both pathways are raised in steatosis, even in non-diabetic patients, contributing to the synthesis of hepatic TG and the promotion of fatty liver. In NAFLD patients the IR promotes the activation of hepatic stellate cells, which are the trigger that initiates the fibrogenesis process that characterize NASH [45]. In the same manner, hepatic synthesis of palmitate (via DNL stimulated by insulin) can cause increases the risk of lipotoxicity and cell damage. Moreover, hyperinsulinemia and IR are considered better predictors of hepatic injury than visceral adiposity [46]. Therefore, insulin high levels and IR conditions are linked with abnormal concentration of lipoproteins, elevated VLDL production, high levels of plasmatic cholesterol, TG and LDL that allows to cardiovascular diseases.

Glucagon

Glucagon function is opposite that of insulin since glucagon stimulates glucose production via activation of hepatic glycogenolysis and gluconeogenesis by glycolysis inhibition. It also regulates fatty acid metabolism via stimulation of peripheral lipolysis, reduction of malonyl-CoA and stimulation of fatty acid oxidation. Elevated plasma concentrations of glucagon have been reported in patients with cirrhosis, chronic hepatitis and fatty liver disease. In this last group, fasting high levels of glucagon were reported whether or not the patients were diabetic [47]. This evidence has suggested that hyperglucagonemia may have originated from a liver-steatosis rather than a pancreatic compensatory signals in the T2D evolution. As in the case of insulin, know if exists a previous hormone-resistance in the tissues, or if the resistance is due to hormonal overstimulation is still the dilemma. However, it was proposed that the level of liver TG may be involved in the mechanism of HF diet-induced glucagon resistance in the liver. This suggestion is supported the TG levels correlated inversely proportional to the glucagon-stimulated hepatic glucose production. Impairment in the expression of glucagon receptors it has been also linked to the liver fat content [48].

Conclusion

A balance between lipid acquisition and disposal establishes intrahepatic fat levels. In general, it has been reported that liver acquires lipids through the uptake of circulating fatty acids (from the diet or adipose tissue lipolysis) and via DNL. Conversely, lipids may be consumed through beta-oxidation ketogenesis and through export VDLD particles. Regarding this, it is possible guess why bariatric surgery is useful in the manage of the fatty liver, since the vast majority of techniques reduces hepatic fat acquisition pathways and regulates IR, common factor in this metabolic disorders.

References

[1] Sarr O, Mathers KE, Zhao L, Dunlop K, Chiu J, Guglielmo CG, et al. Western diet consumption through early life induces microvesicular hepatic steatosis in association with an altered metabolome in low birth weight Guinea pigs. *J Nutr Biochem.* 2019;67:219-33. Epub 2019/04/15. doi: 10.1016/j.jnutbio.2019.02.009. PubMed PMID: 30981986.

[2] Parry SA, Hodson L. Influence of dietary macronutrients on liver fat accumulation and metabolism. *J Investig Med.* 2017;65(8):1102-15. Epub 2017/09/28. doi: 10.1136/jim-2017-000524. PubMed PMID: 28947639; PubMed Central PMCID: PMCPMC5749316.

[3] Saponaro C, Gaggini M, Gastaldelli A. Nonalcoholic fatty liver disease and type 2 diabetes: common pathophysiologic mechanisms. *Curr Diab Rep.* 2015;15(6):607. Epub 2015/04/22. doi: 10.1007/s11892-015-0607-4. PubMed PMID: 25894944.

[4] Chitturi S, Abeygunasekera S, Farrell GC, Holmes-Walker J, Hui JM, Fung C, et al. NASH and insulin resistance: Insulin hypersecretion and specific association with the insulin resistance syndrome. *Hepatology.* 2002;35(2):373-9. Epub 2002/02/05. doi: 10.1053/jhep.2002.30692. PubMed PMID: 11826411.

[5] Lonardo A, Targher G. NAFLD: Is There Anything New under the Sun? *Int J Mol Sci.* 2017;18(9). Epub 2017/09/13. doi: 10.3390/ijms18091955. PubMed PMID: 28895919; PubMed Central PMCID: PMCPMC5618604.

[6] Wattacheril J, Sanyal AJ. Lean NAFLD: An Underrecognized Outlier. *Curr Hepatol Rep.* 2016;15(2):134-9. Epub 2016/09/27. doi: 10.1007/s11901-016-0302-1. PubMed PMID: 27668144; PubMed Central PMCID: PMCPMC5030075.

[7] Stender S, Kozlitina J, Nordestgaard BG, Tybjaerg-Hansen A, Hobbs HH, Cohen JC. Adiposity amplifies the genetic risk of fatty liver disease conferred by multiple loci. *Nat Genet.* 2017;49(6):842-7. Epub 2017/04/25. doi: 10.1038/ng.3855. PubMed PMID: 28436986; PubMed Central PMCID: PMCPMC5562020.

[8] Gastaldelli A. Insulin resistance and reduced metabolic flexibility: cause or consequence of NAFLD? *Clin Sci (Lond).* 2017;131(22): 2701-4. Epub 2017/11/08. doi: 10.1042/CS20170987. PubMed PMID: 29109303.

[9] Nguyen P, Leray V, Diez M, Serisier S, Le Bloc'h J, Siliart B, et al. Liver lipid metabolism. *J Anim Physiol Anim Nutr (Berl).* 2008; 92(3):272-83. Epub 2008/05/15. doi: 10.1111/j.1439-0396.2007.00752.x. PubMed PMID: 18477307.

[10] Ratnayake WM, Galli C. Fat and fatty acid terminology, methods of analysis and fat digestion and metabolism: a background review paper. *Ann Nutr Metab.* 2009;55(1-3):8-43. Epub 2009/09/16. doi: 10.1159/000228994. PubMed PMID: 19752534.

[11] Ipsen DH, Lykkesfeldt J, Tveden-Nyborg P. Molecular mechanisms of hepatic lipid accumulation in non-alcoholic fatty liver disease. *Cell Mol Life Sci.* 2018;75(18):3313-27. Epub 2018/06/25. doi: 10.1007/s00018-018-2860-6. PubMed PMID: 29936596; PubMed Central PMCID: PMCPMC6105174.

[12] Szczepaniak LS, Nurenberg P, Leonard D, Browning JD, Reingold JS, Grundy S, et al. Magnetic resonance spectroscopy to measure hepatic triglyceride content: prevalence of hepatic steatosis in the general population. *Am J Physiol Endocrinol Metab.* 2005;288(2):E462-8.

Epub 2004/09/02. doi: 10.1152/ajpendo.00064.2004. PubMed PMID: 15339742.

[13] Geisler CE, Renquist BJ. Hepatic lipid accumulation: cause and consequence of dysregulated glucoregulatory hormones. *J Endocrinol.* 2017;234(1):R1-R21. Epub 2017/04/22. doi: 10.1530/JOE-16-0513. PubMed PMID: 28428362.

[14] Anton SD, Moehl K, Donahoo WT, Marosi K, Lee SA, Mainous AG, 3rd, et al. Flipping the Metabolic Switch: Understanding and Applying the Health Benefits of Fasting. *Obesity* (Silver Spring). 2018;26(2):254-68. Epub 2017/11/01. doi: 10.1002/oby.22065. PubMed PMID: 29086496; PubMed Central PMCID: PMCPMC5783752.

[15] Cohen JC, Horton JD, Hobbs HH. Human fatty liver disease: old questions and new insights. *Science.* 2011;332(6037):1519-23. Epub 2011/06/28. doi: 10.1126/science.1204265. PubMed PMID: 21700865; PubMed Central PMCID: PMCPMC3229276.

[16] Hodson L, Rosqvist F, Parry SA. The influence of dietary fatty acids on liver fat content and metabolism. Proc Nutr Soc. 2019:1-12. Epub 2019/04/04. doi: 10.1017/S0029665119000569. PubMed PMID: 30942685.

[17] Ngo Sock ET, Le KA, Ith M, Kreis R, Boesch C, Tappy L. Effects of a short-term overfeeding with fructose or glucose in healthy young males. *Br J Nutr.* 2010;103(7):939-43. Epub 2009/11/26. doi: 10.1017/S0007114509992819. PubMed PMID: 19930762.

[18] Tappy L, Le KA, Tran C, Paquot N. Fructose and metabolic diseases: new findings, new questions. *Nutrition.* 2010;26(11-12):1044-9. Epub 2010/05/18. doi: 10.1016/j.nut.2010.02.014. PubMed PMID: 20471804.

[19] Johnston RD, Stephenson MC, Crossland H, Cordon SM, Palcidi E, Cox EF, et al. No difference between high-fructose and high-glucose diets on liver triacylglycerol or biochemistry in healthy overweight men. *Gastroenterology.* 2013;145(5):1016-25 e2. Epub 2013/07/23. doi: 10.1053/j.gastro.2013.07.012. PubMed PMID: 23872500.

[20] Silbernagel G, Lutjohann D, Machann J, Meichsner S, Kantartzis K, Schick F, et al. Cholesterol synthesis is associated with hepatic lipid content and dependent on fructose/glucose intake in healthy humans. *Exp Diabetes Res.* 2012;2012:361863. Epub 2011/12/29. doi: 10.1155/2012/361863. PubMed PMID: 22203835; PubMed Central PMCID: PMCPMC3235776.

[21] Puri P, Baillie RA, Wiest MM, Mirshahi F, Choudhury J, Cheung O, et al. A lipidomic analysis of nonalcoholic fatty liver disease. *Hepatology.* 2007;46(4):1081-90. Epub 2007/07/27. doi: 10.1002/hep.21763. PubMed PMID: 17654743.

[22] Leamy AK, Egnatchik RA, Young JD. Molecular mechanisms and the role of saturated fatty acids in the progression of non-alcoholic fatty liver disease. *Prog Lipid Res.* 2013;52(1):165-74. Epub 2012/11/28. doi: 10.1016/j.plipres.2012.10.004. PubMed PMID: 23178552; PubMed Central PMCID: PMCPMC3868987.

[23] Koopman KE, Caan MW, Nederveen AJ, Pels A, Ackermans MT, Fliers E, et al. Hypercaloric diets with increased meal frequency, but not meal size, increase intrahepatic triglycerides: a randomized controlled trial. *Hepatology.* 2014;60(2):545-53. Epub 2014/03/29. doi: 10.1002/hep.27149. PubMed PMID: 24668862; PubMed Central PMCID: PMCPMC4265261.

[24] Djurhuus CB, Gravholt CH, Nielsen S, Pedersen SB, Moller N, Schmitz O. Additive effects of cortisol and growth hormone on regional and systemic lipolysis in humans. *Am J Physiol Endocrinol Metab.* 2004;286(3):E488-94. Epub 2003/11/06. doi: 10.1152/ajpendo.00199.
2003. PubMed PMID: 14600073.

[25] Watt MJ, Holmes AG, Pinnamaneni SK, Garnham AP, Steinberg GR, Kemp BE, et al. Regulation of HSL serine phosphorylation in skeletal muscle and adipose tissue. *Am J Physiol Endocrinol Metab.* 2006; 290(3):E500-8. Epub 2005/09/29. doi: 10.1152/ajpendo.00361.2005. PubMed PMID: 16188906.

[26] Thorp AA, Schlaich MP. Relevance of Sympathetic Nervous System Activation in Obesity and Metabolic Syndrome. *J Diabetes Res.*

2015;2015:341583. Epub 2015/06/13. doi: 10.1155/2015/341583. PubMed PMID: 26064978; PubMed Central PMCID: PMCPMC4430650.

[27] Wang S, Huang Y, Xu H, Zhu Q, Lu H, Zhang M, et al. Oxidized tea polyphenols prevent lipid accumulation in liver and visceral white adipose tissue in rats. *Eur J Nutr.* 2017;56(6):2037-48. Epub 2016/06/09. doi: 10.1007/s00394-016-1241-x. PubMed PMID: 27271251.

[28] Howe HR, 3rd, Heidal K, Choi MD, Kraus RM, Boyle K, Hickner RC. Increased adipose tissue lipolysis after a 2-week high-fat diet in sedentary overweight/obese men. *Metabolism.* 2011;60(7):976-81. Epub 2010/11/03. doi: 10.1016/j.metabol.2010.09.007. PubMed PMID: 21040937; PubMed Central PMCID: PMCPMC3868457.

[29] Wilson CG, Tran JL, Erion DM, Vera NB, Febbraio M, Weiss EJ. Hepatocyte-Specific Disruption of CD36 Attenuates Fatty Liver and Improves Insulin Sensitivity in HFD-Fed Mice. *Endocrinology.* 2016;157(2):570-85. Epub 2015/12/10. doi: 10.1210/en.2015-1866. PubMed PMID: 26650570; PubMed Central PMCID: PMCPMC4 733118.

[30] Hellerstein MK. De novo lipogenesis in humans: metabolic and regulatory aspects. *Eur J Clin Nutr.* 1999;53 Suppl 1:S53-65. Epub 1999/06/12. PubMed PMID: 10365981.

[31] Sanders FW, Griffin JL. De novo lipogenesis in the liver in health and disease: more than just a shunting yard for glucose. *Biol Rev Camb Philos Soc.* 2016;91(2):452-68. Epub 2015/03/06. doi: 10.1111/brv. 12178. PubMed PMID: 25740151; PubMed Central PMCID: PMCPMC4832395.

[32] Ameer F, Scandiuzzi L, Hasnain S, Kalbacher H, Zaidi N. De novo lipogenesis in health and disease. *Metabolism.* 2014;63(7):895-902. Epub 2014/05/13. doi: 10.1016/j.metabol.2014.04.003. PubMed PMID: 24814684.

[33] Muratoglu M, Kuyumjian J, Kalant N. First-pass hepatic uptake and utilization of glucose in the rat. *Biochem J.* 1986;233(1):245-8. Epub

1986/01/01. doi: 10.1042/bj2330245. PubMed PMID: 3954727; PubMed Central PMCID: PMCPMC1153010.
[34] Basaranoglu M, Basaranoglu G, Sabuncu T, Senturk H. Fructose as a key player in the development of fatty liver disease. *World J Gastroenterol.* 2013;19(8):1166-72. Epub 2013/03/14. doi: 10.3748/wjg.v19.i8.1166. PubMed PMID: 23482247; PubMed Central PMCID: PMCPMC3587472.
[35] Koo HY, Miyashita M, Cho BH, Nakamura MT. Replacing dietary glucose with fructose increases ChREBP activity and SREBP-1 protein in rat liver nucleus. *Biochem Biophys Res Commun.* 2009;390(2):285-9. Epub 2009/10/06. doi: 10.1016/j.bbrc.2009.09.109. PubMed PMID: 19799862.
[36] Amako Y, Munakata T, Kohara M, Siddiqui A, Peers C, Harris M. Hepatitis C virus attenuates mitochondrial lipid beta-oxidation by downregulating mitochondrial trifunctional-protein expression. *J Virol.* 2015;89(8):4092-101. Epub 2015/02/13. doi: 10.1128/JVI.01653-14. PubMed PMID: 25673715; PubMed Central PMCID: PMCPMC4442397.
[37] Mannisto VT, Simonen M, Hyysalo J, Soininen P, Kangas AJ, Kaminska D, et al. Ketone body production is differentially altered in steatosis and non-alcoholic steatohepatitis in obese humans. *Liver Int.* 2015;35(7):1853-61. Epub 2014/12/24. doi: 10.1111/liv.12769. PubMed PMID: 25533197.
[38] Nassir F, Ibdah JA. Role of mitochondria in nonalcoholic fatty liver disease. *Int J Mol Sci.* 2014;15(5):8713-42. Epub 2014/05/20. doi: 10.3390/ijms15058713. PubMed PMID: 24837835; PubMed Central PMCID: PMCPMC4057755.
[39] Geisler CE, Ghimire S, Bogan RL, Renquist BJ. Role of ketone signaling in the hepatic response to fasting. *Am J Physiol Gastrointest Liver Physiol.* 2019;316(5):G623-G31. Epub 2019/02/16. doi: 10.1152/ajpgi.00415.2017. PubMed PMID: 30767679.
[40] Minehira K, Young SG, Villanueva CJ, Yetukuri L, Oresic M, Hellerstein MK, et al. Blocking VLDL secretion causes hepatic steatosis but does not affect peripheral lipid stores or insulin sensitivity

in mice. *J Lipid Res.* 2008;49(9):2038-44. Epub 2008/06/ 03. doi: 10.1194/jlr.M800248-JLR200. PubMed PMID: 18515909; PubMed Central PMCID: PMCPMC3837456.

[41] Lonardo A, Lombardini S, Scaglioni F, Carulli L, Ricchi M, Ganazzi D, et al. Hepatic steatosis and insulin resistance: does etiology make a difference? *J Hepatol.* 2006;44(1):190-6. Epub 2005/09/20. doi: 10.1016/j.jhep.2005.06.018. PubMed PMID: 16168516.

[42] Duvillard L, Florentin E, Pont F, Petit JM, Baillot-Rudoni S, Penfornis A, et al. Endogenous chronic hyperinsulinemia does not increase the production rate of VLDL apolipoprotein B: proof from a kinetic study in patients with insulinoma. *J Clin Endocrinol Metab.* 2011;96(7):2163-70. Epub 2011/03/25. doi: 10.1210/jc.2010-2946. PubMed PMID: 21430026.

[43] Bugianesi E, McCullough AJ, Marchesini G. Insulin resistance: a metabolic pathway to chronic liver disease. Hepatology. 2005; 42(5):987-1000. Epub 2005/10/27. doi: 10.1002/hep.20920. PubMed PMID: 16250043.

[44] Manchanayake J, Chitturi S, Nolan C, Farrell GC. Postprandial hyperinsulinemia is universal in non-diabetic patients with nonalcoholic fatty liver disease. *J Gastroenterol Hepatol.* 2011; 26(3):510-6. Epub 2010/12/16. doi: 10.1111/j.1440-1746.2010. 06528.x. PubMed PMID: 21155882.

[45] Gaggini M, Morelli M, Buzzigoli E, DeFronzo RA, Bugianesi E, Gastaldelli A. Non-alcoholic fatty liver disease (NAFLD) and its connection with insulin resistance, dyslipidemia, atherosclerosis and coronary heart disease. *Nutrients.* 2013;5(5):1544-60. Epub 2013/05/ 15. doi: 10.3390/nu5051544. PubMed PMID: 23666091; PubMed Central PMCID: PMCPMC3708335.

[46] Perseghin G. Lipids in the wrong place: visceral fat and nonalcoholic steatohepatitis. *Diabetes Care.* 2011;34 Suppl 2:S367-70. Epub 2011/05/06. doi: 10.2337/dc11-s249. PubMed PMID: 21525484; PubMed Central PMCID: PMCPMC3632209.

[47] Junker AE, Gluud LL, van Hall G, Holst JJ, Knop FK, Vilsboll T. Effects of glucagon-like peptide-1 on glucagon secretion in patients

with non-alcoholic fatty liver disease. *J Hepatol.* 2016;64(4):908-15. Epub 2015/12/03. doi: 10.1016/j.jhep.2015.11.014. PubMed PMID: 26626496.

[48] Charbonneau A, Unson CG, Lavoie JM. High-fat diet-induced hepatic steatosis reduces glucagon receptor content in rat hepatocytes: potential interaction with acute exercise. *J Physiol.* 2007;579(Pt 1):255-67. Epub 2006/10/21. doi: 10.1113/jphysiol.2006.121954. PubMed PMID: 17053032; PubMed Central PMCID: PMCPMC2075374.

In: Liver Steatosis and Bariatric Surgery ISBN: 978-1-53616-444-2
Editors: Jaime Ruiz-Tovar et al.

Chapter 4

HISTOPATHOLOGY OF NAFLD AND NASH

Soledad García-Gómez-Heras*
Human Histology and Pathology, Health Science Department,
Rey Juan Carlos University, Madrid, Spain

ABSTRACT

The histopathological features of adult NAFLD/NASH are: hepatocellular steatosis, hepatocellular ballooning, inflammatory infiltrate, fibrosis, glycogenated nuclei, apoptotic hepatocytes, Mallory-Denk Bodies (MDBs), iron deposition, megamitochondria and ductular reaction. The necessary components for the diagnosis of NASH are: steatosis (accentuated in zone 3), lobular inflammation (mixed, mild) and hepatocellular ballooning (most apparent near steatotic liver cells, typically in zone 3). Fibrosis is not necessary for the diagnosis of NASH, although it is usually present.

There are different histopathological scoring systems and all have both pros and cons. The methods currently used to semi-quantitatively evaluate the histological lesions of NAFLD are: the NAFLD Activity Score (NAS) and Fibrosis Score by the NASH Clinical Research Network (NASH-CRN) and the 'Fatty Liver Inhibition of Progression (FLIP)' Algorithm

* Corresponding Author's Email: soledad.garcia@urjc.es.

and Steatosis, Activity, and Fibrosis (SAF) Score. These ideas will be, discussed in this chapter.

Keywords: histopathology, NASH, hepatocellular-Steatosis, Mallory-Den bodies, steatohepatitic hepatocellular carcinoma, liver fibrosis

HISTOPHATOLOGICAL LESIONS IN THE LIVER

From a morphological point of view, the liver is an organ with a limited repertoire of responses against aggression. Regardless of the cause, five types of response can be observed.

1. Inflammation

The hepatocyte lesion associated with the arrival of acute or chronic inflammatory cells to the liver is called hepatitis. The attack to liver cells expressing viable antigens by sensitized T lymphocytes is a frequent cause for the hepatic lesion. Inflammation may be limited to the lymphocytes' point of entry (portal spaces) or spread to the rest of parenchyma.

Although hepatocyte necrosis can precede inflammation, it can also be the other way around. When hepatocytes experience necrosis or apoptosis, the macrophages in charge of withdrawing the remainders quickly phagocytize the dead cells and generate groups of inflammatory cells in an otherwise normal parenchyma. Foreign bodies, microorganisms, and different drugs can trigger these granulomatous-type reactions.

2. Degeneration

Alterations that are secondary to toxic or immune aggressions can make hepatocytes adopt a swollen and edematous aspect, ballooning degeneration), with irregular blots in the cytoplasm and huge empty spaces.

Another possibility is when the biliar material retained confers a swollen and diffuse spongy appearance to hepatocytes, vacuolar degeneration.

In viable hepatocytes, different types of substances (like iron, copper, fat or retained biliar material) can accumulate. The concentration of fat droplets inside hepatocytes is called steatosis. When they are multiple tiny droplets that do not displace the nucleus, this is called microvacuolar steatosis, typical of acute alcoholic liver disease, Reye syndrome, and acute hepatic steatosis of pregnancy.

In livers of obese or diabetic patients, a single huge vacuole can be found. It is able to displace the nucleus. This lesion constitutes macrovacuolar steatosis.

3. Cell Death

Any important aggression to the liver can cause hepatocyte destruction.

When cell death is caused by immune or toxic mechanisms, it takes place through apoptosis, in which isolated hepatocytes retract, show pyknosis, and acquire an intensely eosinophilic aspect. Other hepatocytes may swell osmotically and break, in the so-called hydropic degeneration or lithic necrosis.

In the case of necrosis, liver cells appear a bit stained and mummified with a greater frequency due to ischemia (coagulative necrosis).

In the context of ischemia and various pharmacologic and toxic reactions, hepatocellular necrosis is distributed throughout the regions surrounding central veins (centrolobulillar necrosis). Mediozonal or pure periportal necrosis are rare.

In the most severe toxic or inflammatory lesions, apoptosis or necrosis of contiguous hepatocytes may comprehend adjacent lobules following a porto-portal pattern, porto-central pattern, or centro-central pattern (bridging necrosis).

Necroses in whole lobules (submassive necrosis) or in most part of liver parenchyma (massive necrosis) normally cause liver failure.

4. Fibrosis

Tissue generates fibrous tissue as a response to inflammation or to a direct toxic aggression.

This collagen deposit has everlasting consequences for hepatocyte irrigation and perfusion patterns. In the first stages, fibrosis arises in the interior or around porta spaces or central veins, or deposits directly in sinusoids. Over time, fibrous bands end up joining liver regions (porto-portal, porto-central or centro-central). This process is called bridging fibrosis.

Unlike other lesions that are reversible, fibrosis normally is an irreversible consequence of liver lesions. However, under certain circumstances, fibrosis has shown to decrease when the liver lesion has stopped. The best known cases of fibrosis regression are hepatic schistosomiasis infection and hereditary hemochromatosis.

5. Cirrhosis

When fibrosis and parenchymal lesions are maintained, the liver will end up subdivided into nodules of hepatocytes in regeneration, surrounded by scar tissue, and this is called cirrhosis.

It is one of the main causes of death in the Western world. Regardless of etiology, end-stage cirrhosis is characterized by:

- fibrous walls, in the form of delicate bands or wide scars replacing several adjacent lobules.
- parenchymal nodules, caused by the regeneration of hepatocytes that were isolated, of a size ranging from small (less than 3 mm diameter or micronodules) and large (up to several cm diameter or macronodules).
- alteration of the whole liver architecture.

Cirrhosis pathogenesis. The three main anatomopathological mechanisms that combine to produce cirrhosis are hepatocellular death, regeneration, and progressive fibrosis.

Regarding fibrosis, an element to consider is that the normal liver contains types I, III, and IV interstitial collagen. It concentrates in porta spaces and around centrolobulillar veins, with occasional bands in the parenchyma. A delicate reticular grid of IV collagen is arranged in the space between endothelial cells in the sinusoids and hepatocytes (space of Disse). In cirrhosis, type I and III collagen, as well as other components of extracellular matrix, deposit in all portions of lobules, thus causing endothelial cells of the sinusoids to lose their fenestrations. Furthermore, bypasses generate between the porta vein and the liver vein, as well as between the liver artery and the portal vein. All these processes finally transform the sinusoids of fenestrated endothelial channels, where interexchange of solutes between plasma and hepatocytes is free, into vascular channels of a greater pressure and slow flow, in which such solute interexchange does not take place. The impairment is especially marked in the movement of proteins between hepatocytes and plasma.

The greatest part of collagen excess present in cirrhosis seems to come from perisinusoidal Ito cells orstellate cells that store fat and are located in the space of Disse. Although, in normal conditions, their main function is to store vitamin A and lipids, during cirrhosis development they activate and lose their retinol ester deposits and transform into myofibroblastic cells. The stimuli for collagen synthesis and deposit can come from several sources:

- chronic inflammation with synthesis of inflammatory cytokines, TNF, IL-1.
- cytosine production by stimulated endogenous cells (Kupffer cells, endothelial cells, hepatocytes, and epithelial cells in biliary ducts).
- alteration of extracellular matrix.
- direct stimulation of stellate cells by toxins.

TYPICAL NAFLD AND NASH LIVER LESIONS

Histopathologically, non-alcoholic fatty liver disease (NAFLD) is classified into two categories: only hepatocellular steatosis, and nonalcoholic steatohepatitis (NASH), where necroinflammatory damage appears associated with steatosis.

Simple steatosis generally has a benign clinical course, but one third of NAFLD cases progress and advance to NASH, liver cirrhosis and hepatocellular carcinoma (HCC).

The histopathological characteristics of NASH have been established since 2002. The necessary components for the diagnosis of NASH are: steatosis (accentuated in zone 3), lobular inflammation (mixed, mild) and hepatocellular ballooning (most apparent near steatotic liver cells, typically in zone 3). Fibrosis is not necessary for the diagnosis of NASH, although it is usually present.

Most hepatopathologists diagnose NASH according to these criteria, although a complete consensus has not been reached, as we will later explain.

Below are explained the histopathological features of adult NASH. (Figure 1.)

1. Hepatocellular Steatosis

More than 5% of hepatocytes with steatosis is the hallmark of NAFLD.

It is usually macrovesicular, as a single large fat droplet nearly fills or occupies the cytoplasm of hepatocytes, pushing the nucleus to the periphery.

In few cases it can be observed where the cytoplasm of hepatocytes is filled with tiny lipid droplets and the nucleus is located centrally in the cell.

It usually begins in zone 3, and as the diseases progresses, liver affectation extends and becomes severe steatosis. This latter may end up being panacinar steatosis. As the severity of steatosis increases, other accompanying lesions appear as lobular inflammation and zone 3 fibrosis.

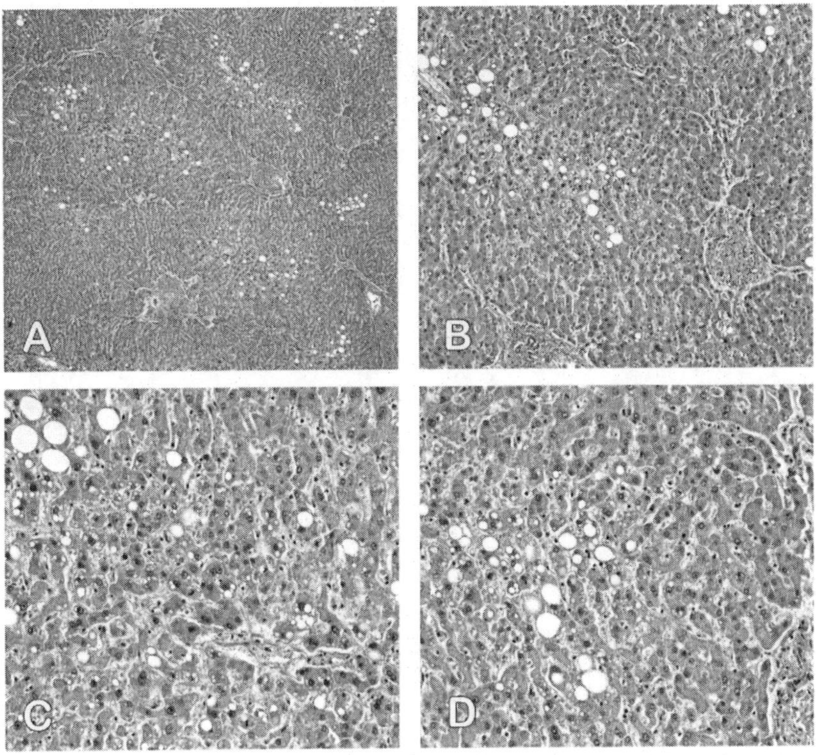

Figure 1. Histopathological lesions in NASH liver. A. hematoxiline-eosin, 100x. B. Portal inflammatory infiltrate. 200x. C and D. Hepatocellular steatosis. 400x.

In cases of panacinar steatosis, it appears associated with ballooning, Mallory-Denk bodies (MDBs) and advanced fibrosis

2. Hepatocellular Ballooning

Ballooning hepatocellular injury is the other key diagnostic feature of steatohepatitis.

This lesion reflects hepatocellular injury. It is characterized as having swollen or "balloon-shaped" hepatocytes that loose the sharp angles and exhibit a clear and non-vacuolar cytoplasm.

These hepatocytes may or may not be larger than non-pathological hepatocytes, fat droplets and/or Mallory-Denk Bodies (MDBs) may be observed in their cytoplasm.

Studies using electron microscopy and immunostaining have evaluated the nature of ballooned hepatocytes. It results from alteration of cytokeratins 8 and 18, the cytoskeleton intermediate filament; they are disrupted and dispersed to the periphery.

In slides stained with hematoxylin and eosin, the recognition of ballooned hepatocytes may be difficult; the loss of cytokeratin 8/18 immunostaining can serve as an objective marker of ballooned hepatocytes.

3. Inflammatory Infiltrate

This can be lobular and portal inflammation.

The lobular inflammation in NASH is usually mild and, when abundant, suggests another or associated causes such as alcohol or drug toxicity.

It consists of a mixed inflammatory cell infiltrate: lymphocytes, neutrophils, eosinophils and Kupffer cells (KC).

It is possible to find an infiltrate predominantly lymphocytary.

Aggregates of neutrophils are rare in NASH and only become prominent around very damaged hepatocytes, and then we can observe ballooned hepatocytes with MDB in the cytoplasm surrounded by neutrophils. This lesion is referred to as "satellitosis". Satellitosis can be occasionally seen in NASH, but is more common in alcoholic hepatitis.

KCs aggregates near sinusoidal capillaries are often found in Nash. They form sparce lobular microgranulomes.

Likewise, lipogranulomas, fat droplets mixed with inflammatory cells and collagen also appear.

Portal inflammation in NAFLD/NASH is usually absent or mild, and consists mainly of lymphocytes. Greater than mild and chronic portal inflammation is associated with the amount and location of steatosis, ballooning and advanced fibrosis Therefore, it could be considered a marker of advanced disease. Finally, when portal inflammation is disproportionately severe, the possibility of concurrence with other liver diseases as hepatitis C or autoimmune hepatitis should be considered.

4. Fibrosis

Fibrosis is a major feature since the stage of fibrosis influences overall and liver related mortality, regardless of the presence or severity of other histological features.

Fibrosis in NASH is observed and associated with an active necroinflammatory reaction. It has a characteristic pattern: perisinusoidal or pericellular and typically begins in zone 3 as a delicate perisinusoidal deposition.

Usually periportal fibrosis develops, with or without zone 3 pericellular fibrosis. In cases of evolution and worsening of the diseases, bridging fibrosis and end-stage cirrhosis appears. In very advanced cases of fibrosis or cirrhosis, steaotosis and necroinflammatory reactions disappear. This state is known as burn-out NASH or cryptogenic cirrhosis.

Particularly in adult NAFLD patients' post-obese intervention, it is possible to see very fine non-zonal sinusoidal fibrosis or any stage of fibrosis without any features of NASH.

NASH-related cirrhosis is most commonly macronodular or mixed.

5. Glycogenated Nuclei

Glycogenated nuclei are vacuolated nuclei observed usually in periportal hepatocytes, and commonly occur in NASH. The presence of glycogenated nuclei is useful for discriminating between NASH and alcoholic steatohepatitis (ASH), as they are rarely observed in ASH.

6. Apoptotic Hepatocytes (Acidophil Bodies)

Often we can observe apoptotic hepatocytes in NASH. These are found in sinusoids as eosinophilic rounded bodies, with hyperchromatic nuclear fragments.

7. Mallory-Denk Bodies (MDBs)

They are eosinophilic irregular-shaped aggregates found in the cytoplasm of hepatocytes.

These structures are usually observed in ballooned hepatocytes in zone 3, and mainly consist of cytokeratins 8 and 18, ubiquitin, and p62.

The presence of MDBs is not definitively required, but is helpful for the diagnosis of NASH. MDBs are not specific to NASH; they are also observed in other liver diseases including chronic cholestasis, HCC and alcoholic hepatitis, where MDBs are also observed in non-ballooned hepatocytes.

8. Iron Deposition

Iron accumulation in NAFLD/NASH is usually mild, and can occur within hepatocytes, the sinusoidal lining cells of the reticuloendothelial system, or both.

The signification of iron deposition in NASH remains unclear. Alenti et al., in 2010, reported that iron accumulation was predominant in hepatocytes and was associated with advanced fibrosis in NASH. However, Nelson et al., in 2011, indicated that NASH patients with iron accumulation in the reticuloendothelial system were more likely to have advanced fibrosis compared to patients with iron accumulation in hepatocytes.

9. Megamitochondria

They are crystal-shaped eosinophilic structures in the cytoplasm of hepatocytes. They may be the result of injury from lipid peroxidation, or could represent an adaptive change.

They are observed most commonly in hepatocytes with microvesicular steatosis. Megamitochondria in NASH are distributed equally in all zones, and are abundant similarly in low- and high-stage groups.

10. Ductular Reaction

This refers to ductular proliferation at the portal tract interface. It arises from progenitor cells in the periportal area, and is accompanied by neutrophils and stromal changes. In NASH, the extent of ductular reaction is associated with fibrosis.

11. Steatohepatitic Hepatocellular Carcinoma (SH-HCC)

NASH can progress to liver cirrhosis and HCC.

However, the pathological features of HCC derived from NASH have not been elucidated.

In 2009, the 5-year incidence of HCC for cirrhotic NASH was reported to be 11.3%.

In 2010, Salomao et al., described a distinctive histological variant of HCC that they termed SH-HCC. SH-HCC shows features that resemble non-neoplastic steatohepatitis, including large droplet steatosis, ballooning of malignant hepatocytes, MDBs, inflammation, and pericellular fibrosis.

In a 2012 study, the same group reported that the prevalence of SH-HCC in all HCC cases was 13.5%. Almost all cases of SH-HCC occurred in patients with underlying steatohepatitis. It was diagnosed in 35.7% of HCC patients with either NASH or alcoholic liver disease, compared with only 1.3% of HCC patients with other chronic liver diseases.

Subsequently, Jain et al. in 2012, reported that SH-HCC was much more common in cirrhotic NASH patients compared with those with alcoholic cirrhosis.

ASSESSMENT SCALES

There are different histopathological scoring systems. All share the assessment of four histological lesions: extent of steatosis, grade of inflammation, hepatocyte ballooning, and staging of fibrosis. All have both pros and cons which will be discussed here.

The methods currently used to semi-quantitatively evaluate the histological lesions of NAFLD and to cover the spectrum of the disease are:

- the NAFLD Activity Score (NAS) and Fibrosis Score by the NASH Clinical Research Network (NASH-CRN).
- the 'Fatty Liver Inhibition of Progression (FLIP)' Algorithm and Steatosis, Activity, and Fibrosis (SAF) Score.

The first scale proposed by Brunt et al. in 1999 was purely histological.

In 1999, there were no systems for grading necroinflammatory activity or fibrosis as did exist for various other forms of chronic liver disease. Brunt EM et al., wanted to develop such a grading system. After the revision of liver biopsies from patients with nonalcoholic steatohepatitis from Saint Louis University Health Sciences Center, they concluded that histological lesions considered to be significant were: steatosis, ballooning, and intra-acinar and portal inflammation. They developed a staging score where they classified the necroinflammatory grades of NASH as grade 1 (mild), grade 2 (moderate), and grade 3 (severe) based on the degree of hepatocellular steatosis, ballooning and inflammation (intralobular and portal). (Table 1). The range is from 0 to 8.

Steatosis grade ranges 0 to 3, where normal liver (grade 0) contains fat in < 5% of hepatocytes, and grade 1, grade 2, and grade 3 steatosis refer to at least 5%, 33%, or 66% of steatotic hepatocytes, respectively.

Lobular inflammation is graded 0 to 3 based on the number of inflammatory foci in a given area.

Grading of ballooning ranges 0 to 2 and is mainly based on the number of ballooned hepatocytes.

Table 1. NAFLD/NASH Scale proposed by Brunt et al. in 1999

GRADING	Grade 1 (MILD)	Steatosis up to 66%
		Ballooning: occasional in zone 3
		Intralobular inflammation: scattered polymorphs ± lymphocytes
		Portal inflammation: no or mild
	Grade 2 (MODERATE)	Steatosis: any degree
		Ballooning: obvious, predominantly zone 3
		Intralobular inflammation: polymorphs and chronic inflammation noted
		Portal inflammation: mild to moderate
	Grade 3 (SEVERE)	Steatosis: panacinar
		Ballooning: ballooning and disarray obvious, predominantly in zone 3
		Intralobular inflammation: scattered polymorphs ± mild chronic inflammation
		Portal inflammation: mild or moderate.
STAGING	Stage 1	Zone 3 perisinusoidal/pericellular fibrosis, focal or extensive
	Stage 2	Zone 3 perisinusoidal/pericellular fibrosis + focal or extensive periportal fibrosis
	Stage 3	Zone 3 perisinusoidal/pericellular fibrosis + portal fibrosis + bridging fibrosis
	Stage 4	Cirrhosis

For staging and quantifying liver fibrosis based on the location and extent of fibrosis, the scoring system is: stage 1, zone 3 perisinusoidal fibrosis; stage 2, portal fibrosis with the abovementioned stage 1; stage 3, bridging fibrosis in addition to stage 2; and stage 4, cirrhosis.

In 2005, The NASH Clinical Research Network (NASH CRN) designed and validated the histological NAFLD Activity Score (NAS) scoring system that addresses the full spectrum of NAFLD/NASH lesions. (Table 2).

It is based on the notion in liver disease that the necroinflammatory lesions and the stage of fibrosis should be separately evaluated because the former are potentially more reversible than the latter.

Table 2. NAFLD/NASH Scale propsed in 2005 by The NASH Clinical Research Network (NASH CRN)

NAFLD ACTIVITY SCORE(NAS) and FIBROSIS SCORE By the CLINICAL RESEARCH NETWORK (NASH-CNR)			**POINTS**
	Steatosis(S)	< 5%	0
		5 - 33%	1
		34 - 66%	2
		> 66%	3
	Lobular Inflammation(Ll)	0	0
		< 2/20x	1
		2 - 4/20x	2
		> 4/20x	3
	Ballooning (B)	None	0
		Few	1
		Many	2
	Fibrosis Stage(F)	None	0
		Zone 3 perisinusoidal, delicate	1a
		Zone 3 perisinusoidal, dense	1b
		Portal only	1c
		1^{a} or 1b + portal	2
		bridging	3
		Cirrhosis	4
SCORES	**NAS: S + Ll + B = 0 - 8**		

Based on Brunt, they classified the necroinflammatory grades of NASH as grade 1 (mild), grade 2 (moderate), and grade 3 (severe) according to the degree of hepatocellular steatosis, ballooning and inflammation (intralobular and portal).

NASH CRN subclassified Bunt stage 1 into 3 categories: stage 1A, mild perisinusoidal fibrosis in zone 3; stage 1B, moderate perisinusoidal fibrosis in zone 3; and stage 1C, only portal/periportal fibrosis. Stage 1C fibrosis is observed occasionally in children or severely obese patients.

Currently, the NAS is one of the most widely used histological classifications for NAFLD/NASH and its use is recommended for defining and quantifying disease activity in observational and interventional trials of NAFLD/NASH.

But, accumulating evidence indicates that the NAS is poorly correlated with metabolic risk factors and is unable to predict both the risk of fibrosis progression [and (liver-related and overall) mortality in NAFLD.

In 2012, Bedossa et al., wanted to build an algorithm along with a scoring system for histopathologic classification of liver lesions that covered the entire spectrum of lesions in morbidly obese patients.

They suggest that the SAF score evaluates the grade of steatosis (S), the grade of activity (A), and the stage of fibrosis (F). The A grade (A0 to A4) is computed by adding grades of ballooning to lobular inflammation.

They built an algorithm for the histopathological lesions segregating lesions into normal liver, NAFLD, or nonalcoholic steatohepatitis (NASH) based on semiquantitative evaluation of steatosis, hepatocellular ballooning, and lobular inflammation. For each case, the SAF score was created including the semiquantitative scoring of steatosis (S), activity (A), and fibrosis (F).

Compared to the NAS score, the SAF scores the grading of hepatocellular ballooning based chiefly on both size and shape of ballooned hepatocytes.

At variance with the NAS, the SAF score does not include steatosis in the activity score. The philosophy behind this is that, compared to hepatocellular ballooning and lobular inflammation, steatosis *per se* is an arguable prognostic marker of disease progression. Moreover, the fibrosis stage, although an acknowledged outcome modifier in chronic liver disease owing to various etiologies, is not part of NAS.

The SAF score allows for the definition of categories of NAFLD severity (mild disease when $A < 2$ and $F < 2$ vs. significant disease when $A \geq 2$ and/or $F \geq 2$), defined by hepatocellular ballooning, lobular inflammation, and fibrosis, that is, those parameters of recognized prognostic significance in NAFLD.

Table 3. NAFLD/NASH Scale proposed by European FLIP (Fatty Liver Inhibition of Progression Consortium) in 2014

SAF/FLIP ALGORITHM			POINTS
	Steatosis(S)	< 5%	0
		5 - 33%	1
		34 - 66%	2
		> 66%	3
	Lobular Inflammation(Ll)	0	0
		< 2/20x	1
		2 - 4/20x	2
		-	-
	Ballooning (B)	None	0
		Clusters, reticulated cytoplasm	1
		Enlarged hepatocytes	2
	Fibrosis Stage(F)	None	0
		Zone 3 perisinusoidal, (all), or portal only	1
		Zona 3 + periportal	2
		-	-
		-	-
		bridging	3
		Cirrhosis	4
SCORES	**SAF: S + ACTIVITY(A: Ll + B) + FIBROSIS = S0 - 3 A0 - 4 F0 - 4**		

In 2014, the European FLIP (Fatty Liver Inhibition of Progression Consortium) designed the FLIP algorithm based on the SAF score to decrease interobserver variations among pathologists and to be implemented in pathology practice. The aim of this study was to determine whether the use of the SAF score and FLIP algorithm can decrease interobserver variations among pathologists. The FLIP algorithm based on the SAF score should decrease interobserver variations among pathologists and is likely to be implemented in pathology practice.

The FLIP algorithm (Table 3) is based on semi-quantitation of the three elementary liver histological features. Steatosis is graded 0 to 3, ballooning 0 to 2, and lobular inflammation 0 to 2.

The FLIP algorithm aims at enabling a binary classification: NASH as opposed to "steatosis without NASH". NASH is diagnosed based on the combination of all three elementary histological features provided that each of these three features has a grade ≥ 1.

Differential Diagnosis between NASH and Other Diseases Affecting the Liver

After a complete and detailed medical history, obviously taking into account clinical information regarding alcohol intake, a differential diagnosis with the following diseases should be made:

- alcoholic liver disease (ASH).
- drug-induced liver injury.
- Wilson's disease.
- α1-antitrypsin deficiency.
- viral hepatitis.

From a histological point of view, the differential diagnosis between NASH and ASH is the most frequent. The main differences with ASH are:

1. Features that are more common in NASH than ASH include severe steatosis, glycogenated nuclei, and lipogranulomas. Fibrosis in NASH shows a lattice pattern.
2. Histological features more common in ASH than NASH include:
    - Canalicular cholestasis.
    - MDBs in ASH are numerous and well formed.

- A prominent ductular reaction.
- Acute inflammation and fibrosis in the portal tract.
- Fibrosis in alcoholic liver disease shows a solid pattern on reticulin-stained slides.
- Necroinflammatory activity in ASH is more severe than in NASH.
- Sclerosing hyaline necrosis and veno-occlusive lesions are observed occasionally in alcoholic liver disease, but these lesions have not been reported in NAFLD.

References

Alenti, L; Fracanzani, AL; Bugianesi, E; Dongiovanni, P; Galmozzi, E; Vanni, E; Canavesi, E; Lattuada, E; Roviaro, G; Marchesini, G; Fargion, S. "HFE genotype, parenchymal iron accumulation, and liver fibrosis in patients with nonalcoholic fatty liver disease". *Gastroenterology.*, 2010, 138, 905-912.

Angulo, P; Kleiner, DE; Dam-Larsen, S; et al. "Liver fibrosis, but no other histologic features; is associated with long-term outcomes of patients with nonalcoholic fatty liver disease". *Gastroenterology.*, 2015, 149, 389–97.

Ballestri, S; Nascimbeni, F; Romagnoli, D; et al. "The independent predictors of non-alcoholic steatohepatitis and its individual histological features: insulin resistance, serum uric acid, metabolic syndrome, alanine aminotransferase and serum total cholesterol are a clue to pathogenesis and candidate targets for treatment". *Hepatol Res.*, 2016, 46, 1074–1087.

Bedossa, P; Poitou, C; Veyrie, N; et al. "Histopathological algorithm and scoring system for evaluation of liver lesions in morbidly obese patients". *Hepatology.*, 2012, 56, 1751–1759.

Bedossa, P; Consortium, FP. "Utility and appropriateness of the fatty liver inhibition of progression (FLIP) algorithm and steatosis, activity, and fibrosis (SAF) score in the evaluation of biopsies of nonalcoholic fatty liver disease". *Hepatology.*, 2014, 60, 565–575.

Bedossa, P. "Pathology of non-alcoholic fatty liver disease". *Liver International*, 2017, 37, (Suppl. 1), 85–89.

Brunt, EM; Janney, CG; Di Bisceglie, AM; NeuschwanderTetri, BA; Bacon, BR. "Nonalcoholic steatohepatitis: a proposal for grading and staging the histological lesions". *Am J Gastroenterol*, 1999, 94, 2467-2474.

Brunt, EM; Tiniakos, DG. "Alcoholic and non-alcoholic fatty liver disease". In: Odze RD, Goldblum JR, Crawford JM. *Pathology of the GI tract, liver, biliary tract and pancreas*. Philadelphia. Ed Saunders, 2009, 1087-1114.

Brunt, EM; Tiniakos, DG. "Histopathology of nonalcoholic fatty liver disease". *World J Gastroenterol*, 2010, 16, 5286-5296.

Brunt, EM. "Non-alcoholic fatty liver disease: what's new under the microscope?" *Gut*, 2011, 60, 1152-1158.

Brunt, E; Kleiner, D; Wilson, L; Belt, P; Neuschwander, B." The NAS and The Histopathologic Diagnosis in NAFLD: Distinct Clinicopathologic Meanings". *Hepatology.*, 2011, 53(3), 810–820.

Brunt, EM; Kleiner, DE; Wilson, LA; et al. "Nonalcoholic fatty liver disease (NAFLD) activity score and the histopathologic diagnosis in NAFLD: distinct clinicopathologic meanings". *Hepatology.*, 2011, 53, 810–820.

Cohen, JC; Horton, JD; Hobbs, HH. "Human fatty liver disease: old questions and new insights". *Science*, 2011, 332, 1519-1523.

Ekstedt, M; Franzen, LE; Mathiesen, UL; et al. "Low clinical relevance of the nonalcoholic fatty liver disease activity score (NAS) in predicting fibrosis progression" *Scand J Gastroenterol.*, 2012, 47, 108–115.

Ekstedt, M; Hagstrom, H; Nasr, P; et al. "Fibrosis stage is the strongest predictor for disease-specific mortality in NAFLD after up to 33 years of follow-up". *Hepatology.*, 2015, 61, 1547–1554.

Feldstein, AE; Gores, GJ. Apoptosis in alcoholic and nonalcoholic steatohepatitis. *Front Biosci.*, 2005, 10, 3093-3099.

Jain, D; Nayak, NC; Saigal, S. "Hepatocellular carcinoma in nonalcoholic fatty liver cirrhosis and alcoholic cirrhosis: risk factor analysis in liver transplant recipients". *Eur J Gastroenterol Hepatol*, 2012, 24, 840-848.

Kleiner, DE; Brunt, EM; Van Natta, M; et al. "Design and validation of a histological scoring system for nonalcoholic fatty liver disease". *Hepatology.*, 2005, 41, 1313–1321, 21.

Le, TH; Caldwell, SH; Redick, JA; Sheppard, BL; Davis, CA; Arseneau, KO; Iezzoni, JC; Hespenheide, EE; Al-Osaimi, A; Peterson, TC. "The zonal distribution of megamitochondria with crystalline inclusions in nonalcoholic steatohepatitis." *Hepatology.*, 2004, 39, 1423-1429.

Nakano, M; Fukusato, T. "Histological study on comparison between NASH and ALD". *Hepatol Res.*, 2005, 33, 110-115.

Nelson, JE; Wilson, L; Brunt, EM; Yeh, MM; Kleiner, DE; Unalp-Arida, A; Kowdley, KV. "Relationship between the pattern of hepatic iron deposition and histological severity in nonalcoholic fatty liver disease." *Hepatology*, 2011, 53, 448-457.

Neuschwander-Tetri, BA; Caldwell, SH. "Nonalcoholic steatohepatitis: summary of an AASLD Single Topic Conference". *Hepatology*, 2003, 37, 1202-1219.

Ong, J; Younossi, ZM; Reddy, V; Price, LL; Gramlich, T; Mayes, J; Boparai, N. Cryptogenic cirrhosis and posttransplantation nonalcoholic fatty liver disease. *Liver Transpl*, 2001, 7, 797-801.

Pinto, HC; Baptista, A; Camilo, ME; Valente, A; Saragoça, A; de Moura, MC. "Nonalcoholic steatohepatitis. Clinicopathological comparison with alcoholic hepatitis in ambulatory and hospitalized patients". *Dig Dis Sci.*, 1996, 41, 172-179.

Richardson, MM; Jonsson, JR; Powell, EE; Brunt, EM; Neuschwander-Tetri, BA; Bhathal, PS; Dixon, JB; Weltman, MD; Tilg, H; Moschen, AR; Purdie, DM; Demetris, AJ; Clouston, AD. "Progressive fibrosis in nonalcoholic steatohepatitis: association with altered regeneration and a ductular reaction". *Gastroenterology*, 2007, 133, 80-90.

Salomao, M; Yu, WM; Brown, RS; Emond, JC; Lefkowitch, JH. "Steatohepatitic hepatocellular carcinoma (SH-HCC): a distinctive histological variant of HCC in hepatitis C virus related cirrhosis with associated NAFLD/NASH". *Am J Surg Pathol*, 2010, 34, 1630-1636.

Salomao, M; Remotti, H; Vaughan, R; Siegel, AB; Lefkowitch, JH; Moreira, RK. "The steatohepatitic variant of hepatocellular carcinoma and its association with underlying steatohepatitis". *Hum Pathol.*, 2012, 43, 737-746.

Skoien, R; Richardson, MM; Jonsson, JR; Powell, EE; Brunt, EM; et al. Heterogeneity of fibrosis patterns in non-alcoholic fatty liver disease supports the presence of multiple fibrogenic pathways". *Liver Int*, 2013, 33, 624-632.

Tiniakos, DG. Nonalcoholic fatty liver disease/nonalcoholic steatohepatitis: histological diagnostic criteria and scoring systems. *Eur J Gastroenterol Hepatol*, 2010, 22, 643-650.

Yatsuji, S; Hashimoto, E; Tobari, M; Taniai, M; Tokushige, K; Shiratori, K. "Clinical features and outcomes of cirrhosis due to non-alcoholic steatohepatitis compared with cirrhosis caused by chronic hepatitis C". *J Gastroenterol Hepatol*, 2009, 24, 248-254.

Younossi, ZM; Reddy, V; Price, LL; Gramlich, T; Mayes, J; Boparai, N. "Cryptogenic cirrhosis and posttransplantation nonalcoholic fatty liver disease". *Liver Transpl*, 2001, 7, 797-801.

Younossi, ZM; Stepanova, M; Rafiq, N; et al. "Pathologic criteria for nonalcoholic steatohepatitis, interprotocol agreement and ability to predict liver-related mortality". *Hepatology.*, 2011, 53, 1874–1882.

Yoshihisa, T; Fukusato, T. "Histopathology of nonalcoholic fatty liver disease/nonalcoholic steatohepatitis". *World J Gastroenterol.*, 2014, 20(42), 15539-15548.

Zatloukal, K; French, SW; Stumptner, C; Strnad, P; Harada, M; Toivola, DM; Cadrin, M; Omary, MB. "From Mallory to Mallory-Denk bodies: what, how and why?" *Exp Cell Res*, 2007, 313, 2033-2049.

In: Liver Steatosis and Bariatric Surgery ISBN: 978-1-53616-444-2
Editors: Jaime Ruiz-Tovar et al.

Chapter 5

LIVER BIOPSY AS THE "GOLD STANDARD" IN NASH DIAGNOSIS

Soledad García-Gómez-Heras**, MD, PhD,
Raquel Franco-Rodríguez, and Julio Paredes-González
Human Histology and Pathology, Health Science Department,
Rey Juan Carlos University, Madrid, Spain

ABSTRACT

Liver biopsy is the "gold standard" for the diagnosis and evaluation of NAFLD/NASH disease. It is an invasive procedure but we can confirm, characterize the severity of parenchymal changes, and distinguish between NAFLD, steatohepatitis and NASH, associated with the progression of liver injury. Also, it provides a semi-quantitative evaluation of the severity of injuries (Assessment Scales), extremely useful in clinical trials.

The histological and anatomopathological study is a set of procedures fully used both for diagnoses and for investigation. Such procedures require meticulous care in their elaboration due to the sensitivity of these techniques. The different steps in the processing of the tissue are explained in this chapter.

* Corresponding Author's Email: soledad.garcia@urjc.es.

Keywords: liver biopsy, diagnosis, histopathology, NASH, NAFLD, gold-standard

Introduction

Liver biopsy is the "gold standard" for the diagnosis and evaluation of NAFLD/NASH disease. The histopathological evaluation of liver biopsy samples remains central in a patient with clinical signs of NAFLD to exclude other causes of chronic liver disease, to confirm or to exclude the diagnosis of NAFDL/NASH, to evaluate the severity if it is confirmed and to demonstrate if patients have cirrhosis.

Advantages of Liver Biospsy

Liver biopsy plays a unique role compared to non-invasive assessments; thanks to the biopsy we can confirm and characterize the severity of parenchymal changes, distinguish between NAFL, processes that are considered to be slowly progressive, and steatohepatitis, NASH, associated with the progression of liver injury. Also, it provides a semi-quantitative evaluation of the severity of injuries (Assessment Scales, see below), extremely useful in clinical trials.

None of the non-invasive techniques tests can determine if liver injury and fibrosis is really due to NAFLD or to another coexistent liver disorder. On the one hand, nor ultrasound nor computerized tomography (CT) can determine if patients actually have NASH.

On the other hand, elastography and magnetic resonance imaging (MRI) attempt to diagnose NASH base on the assessment of fibrosis and presume that patients with suspected NAFLD and fibrosis have NASH.

Disadvantages of Liver Biospsy

It is an invasive procedure, which requires hospitalization in nearly 3% of cases and is complicated by a 0.3% mortality.

Liver biopsy does have risk of clinical complications, small but real, including:

- pneumothorax.
- pain.
- significant bleeding, 0.3% of persons with a normal platelet count and normal levels of clotting factors.

Additionally, the histopathological NAFLD liver lesions are not uniformly distributed; the liver is not affected homogenously ans as the size of biospsy sample represents a small fraction of the entire organ, the significance of the sample is a subject that should be taken into account.

Because all the above, liver biopsy cannot be considered as a screening procedure in high-risk patient populations; liver biopsy is also unsuitable in long-term monitoring of patients with NAFLD and assessing their response to therapy. Thus, it should definitely be restricted only to those patients who have a high probability of significant liver fibrosis.

Gunn et al. proposed that a liver biopsy should be performed in the following cases:

- All features of metabolic syndrome and obesity.
- T2DM and elevated liver transaminases.
- Normal BMI with elevated liver transaminases
- Elastography greater than 6 kPa.
- Elevated value with a fibrosis scoring system.
- Reliable elastography value cannot be obtained because of obesity.
- Patients are not motivated to lose weight.

And a deferred Liver biopsy when:

- Two or fewer features of metabolic syndrome.
- Normal liver transaminases and absence of T2DM.
- Elastography less than 6 kPa.
- Low value with a fibrosis scoring system.
- Patients are motivated to lose weight.

Processing of Liver Samples Obtained by Biopsy

The histological and anatomopathological study allows us to observe tissues and their different structures, the cells that make it up, and even their ultra-structure through a set of techniques called histological techniques. This set of procedures is fully used both for diagnoses and for investigation. Such procedures require meticulous care in their elaboration due to the sensitivity of these techniques. Therefore, one needs to be aware that an incorrect procedure in any of these steps will produce an altered image that could lead to incorrect results.

Biopsy Types

Samples for the histological study come from biopsies. The biopsy is a surgical procedure from which a small cell tissue sample is obtained from a lesion, tissue or organ for subsequent processing and study under a microscope. Depending on the amount of extracted material and the method used, biopsies can be classified in several types:

1. Incisional Biopsy

Incisional biopsy is that in which only a piece of tissue, mass, or tumor is surgically obtained. Two additional types can be found inside this category:

- *percutaneous biopsy.* The sample is obtained by introducing a needle into the tissue or lesion. The result is a tissue cylinder whose thickness depends on the needle's gauge. Based on the gauge, they are classified in FNAB (fine-needle aspiration biopsy) or CNB (core-needle biopsy).
- *endoscopic biopsy.* The sample is obtained using an endoscope, which is a thin flexible tube that has a light source and a camera at one end. This camera relays high resolution images of the studied site to a television screen.

2. Excisional Biopsy

Excisional biopsy is that in which a full organ, tumor or lesion is surgically obtained.

In this chapter, we will focus on liver biopsy. The study target and source for the samples in this biopsy is the liver. Sampling takes place through percutaneous biopsy, transvenous and/or laparoscopic biopsy.

Percutaneous liver biopsy is the most used. It involves the introduction of a thin needle through the abdomen to reach the liver in order to draw a sample. The sampling is assisted by imaging methods, such as echography or computed tomography. Two types of needles are used for the liver puncture, thus generating two different hepatic cylinders. In one of them, the cylinder is obtained by means of the cut, as with Trucut or Vin Vilverman needles; in the other by means of suction, as with Menghini, Klatskin or Jamshidi needles. In recent years, a new type of automatic needle for biopsies has been developed. This is Trucut-type needles for trimming, which do not need manual handling.

Transvenous liver biopsy takes place by introducing, through the jugular vein, a specially designed hollow tube that allows for the introduction, inside of it, of a biopsy needle, as well as for the extraction of tissue samples when the liver is reached.

Laparoscopic liver biopsy is guided by a laparoscope, which is a flexible tube that has a light and a camera. It is introduced in the abdominal cavity through small incisions. Air is then inserted into the cavity leaving an observation and working area, in order to monitor the liver state on the surface, and to take samples in areas of interest.

Processing of the Tissue (Figure 1)

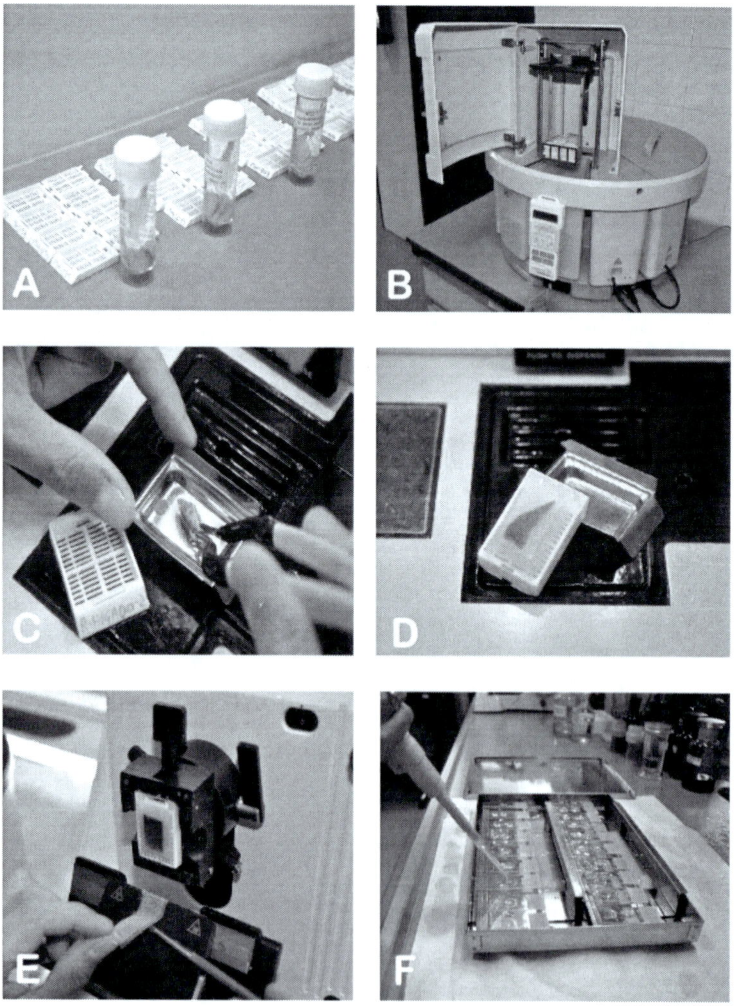

Figure 1. The steps in the processing of liver samples obtained through biopsy. A. Fixation. B. Paraffin embedding. C. and D. Block preparation. E. Obtention of tissue cuts with a minot-type microtome. F. Staining the samples.

I. Fixation

Whatever the means of obtaining the tissue sample, the first step after obtaining the sample is the sample fixation process. This is of vital importance, because it will be a determinant for good development of the other procedures. With this process, we intend to preserve the tissue for study in a state as close as possible to what it was when it was in vivo. To do this, we need to prevent cell autolysis and to stop enzymatic processes. We also have to avoid the action of bacteria, which would start putrefaction processes. And, at the same time, we also want to provide the sample with the hardness necessary for handling it easily, and for its posterior sectioning process.

In order to have the sample fixed correctly and efficiently, the following premises should be taken into account:

- The tissue must come into contact with the fixation agent as soon as possible. The best way to do this is to make a perfusion. To do so, liquid fixative is introduced into the circulating system so that it reaches the tissue. Obviously, such process is not possible in a hospital biopsy, and is normally more used in test animals.
- The volume of liquid fixative should be ten to twenty times greater than the volume of the sample, in order to let it work more efficiently. The fixative is recommended to be at a temperature of 4ºC-5ºC. The sample must be free of blood, mucus, or any other product that could hinder the liquid fixative's penetration into the tissue. Therefore, it is recommended to rinse the sample with physiological or buffered saline solution (in order to prevent an osmotic imbalance from damaging the specimen). Likewise, the liquid fixative used should have an osmotic balance with the sample. To be sure, saline solutions can be used as a solvent for the fixation agent.
- Sample size. The type of tissue should also be born in mind. If we are going to work with a compact or lax tissue, the liquid fixation agent will be able to penetrate with more or less ease. If the tissue presents membranes hampering the fixative's introduction, and of

course, the thickness of the sample: it is always recommended to have a thin sample with edges being as flat as possible.

- The fixative should not cause any alterations in the tissue, such as retractions or swelling, or any change that could affect its morphology. Any variations introduced in the tissue, should be in order to make the posterior handling of the piece easier, or to improve its tinctorial strength.
- The specimen's fixation time must be optimal. It is not recommended to leave the tissue in the fixation agent too long or, obviously, too little time. The optimal time depends on the type of fixative or the fixative mixture used. Each one has an ideal fixation time, which should be followed.

There are several ways to classify fixatives. One of the main ways is depending on whether they act physically or chemically on the tissue. *Fixation through physical processes* takes place by freezing the tissue. This method presents advantages and disadvantages. The main advantage is speed and wide conservation of antigens, enzymes, and proteins, which makes it a very useful fixation for intraoperative biopsies, and for histochemical and immunohistochemical techniques. Some of its weaknesses are the short durability of the samples, the need for expensive frozen storage systems, the huge risk of breaking tissue structures during the freezing process despite using buffered solutions to prevent the formation of crystals in the cells, etc. The most widely used substances for freezing are liquid nitrogen and isopentane at -50ºC, which is the most commonly used for cryodesiccation and cryosubstitution.

Tissue *fixation through chemical processes* takes place through chemical substances that are normally used in an aqueous solution. They act on the tissue by stabilizing it and stopping its processes, while they also act as a bactericide to preserve it. They can be classified as simple or compound fixatives, based on the amount of substances that comprise them: just one or several.

They can also be classified according to how they act on the tissue.

Some fixatives act by dehydrating tissue. They generate protein denaturing, leading to a quick outflow of water from the tissue structures. Some examples are methanol, chloroform, ethanol and acetone.

There are also fixatives whose action takes place through *salt formation*. These normally have a great capacity to penetrate the tissue, and these fixatives spread throughout tissues at a rapid pace. But, at the same time, they present the disadvantage that the formation of those salts creates a crust on the sample, thus minimizing penetration. Therefore, they are normally adequate to be used in fixation mixtures, but are rarely used individually. Examples of these fixatives are mercury chloride or "corrosive sublimate", which is very often used for hematopoietic pathologies, potassium dichromate, which is very good for preparing tissues for silver impregnation techniques, or the picric acid, which is useful as it does not dissolve fat or glycogen, and has a slight decalcification action.

Others take action through *protein reticularization.* They generate protein denaturation, in which hydrogen bridges break, and a reticular polypeptide net is generated. Formaldehyde and formol, with all their variations, glutaraldehyde or osmium tetroxide, which are used in electronic microscopy techniques, are some of the fixatives in this group.

Since *formaldehyde and formol* are part of the most used fixatives, their advantages and disadvantages will be discussed a bit deeper. Formol is used so frequently because of its versatility for fixing all tissue structures. Its tissue penetration rate is not as rapid as other fixatives acting through dehydration, but it still is well above fixatives acting by forming salts. It performs very well as a bactericide and causes almost no tissue alteration phenomena, such as retraction or an excessive hardening. It is effective for the fixation of lipid structures, and normally leaves no deposits in the tissue nor does it interfere with posterior staining. It is very affordable, and can be used both as a single fixation agent, and in fixative mixtures. Its main disadvantages include irritating vapors and its current classification by the European Parliament as a carcinogen category 1B and mutagen category 2. Therefore, it must always be used with all protection measures available. It is also unstable when exposed to sunlight and the atmosphere. If the pH of the formol dissolution decreases below 6, crystals called formolic pigments may start depositing in the tissues, thus altering the posterior staining image. In order to solve these stability problems, the pH, and to improve any issues that could arise due to osmotic differences with the sample, formol 4% is normally used in a buffer solution such as a phosphate, which we call buffered formol.

Finally, there are *fixatives that act through changes in the colloidal state*. They decrease the pH of colloidal solutions where there are proteins and make them precipitate. Among them, we find acetic acid, which preserves nucleoproteins and nucleic acids well, and chromic acid, which is an excellent structural fixative, and acts as mordant of the tissue in stainings where basic coloring will be used.

Regarding *fixative mixtures*, they can be divided into formol-containing or formol-free mixtures. Below, some examples are listed. Among the fixative mixtures with formol, the following can be found:

- *Bouin's solution:* its fixation time goes from 4 to 24 hours, depending on the sample thickness. It requires posterior washes in ethanol at 80% until picric acid remnants are removed. It requires special attention to prevent the piece from hardening too much due to the successive washes in ethanol. It is recommended to include the sample immediately after that. This fixation is efficient in embryonic or testicular samples, and acts as mordent in techniques such as Masson's trichrome staining. However, it is discouraged in kidney samples, due to the alterations generated in the resulting image.
- *Ciaccio's fixative:* its fixation time is 48 hours, and after that, a wash under running water for 24 hours is required. Using this fixative is recommended for lipid tissues or with high fat content.
- *Susa-Heidenhain mixture:* its fixation time goes from 1 to 12 hours. After that time, samples require washes in ethanol 80%. Afterwards, they can be preserved in ethanol 70% for a while. This mixture presents a slight decalcification power.

Among the fixative mixtures that contain no formol, are the following:

- *Carnoy's solution:* This mixture has a maximum fixture time of 2 hours, due to its great capacity for penetrating tissues. Afterwards, samples must be washed with absolute ethanol. Apart from the fixation process, this mixture also acts as sample dehydrating, leaving this step ready for posterior inclusion. It is a much recommended fixation to preserve nucleic acids, Nissl lumps, fibrillary proteins, myofibrilles, and glycogen.
- *Zenker's fixative:* This mixture requires a solution made at the time of use. Its maximum fixation time goes from 2 to 48 hours. Samples fixed in Zenker, once cut and deparaffinized, need to undergo a process called dezenkering. This involves treating the sample with an iodized solution, and then with a sodium thiosulfate solution to remove residues that mercury salts leave on the tissue. This fixation is much used for bone marrow and other hematopoietic tissues, as well as for lymphoid tissue, due to the good preservation of nuclei. It also acts as a mordent in some stainings, such as the phosphotungstic acid-hematoxylin stain.

We would also like to mention the fixation patterns that require histological techniques such as *electron microscopy*. Samples for transmission or scanning electron microscopy need a fixation according to the special needs required for the observation of samples at such magnifications and the particular workings of these microscopes. In these cases, a double or triple fixation is used. The first agent normally is a fixative belonging to the aldehyde family (glutaraldehyde is the most frequently used), although formaldehyde or even other types of fixatives such as potassium permanganate or uranyl acetate can also be used. Based on the ultra-structures that we want to observe, some fixatives will be more adequate than others. It is of vital importance that the fixative be in a buffer solution favoring a stable pH, with no changes in the sample's osmolarity, and that it have an appropriate ionic constitution so as to prevent the cell components from being extracted or precipitate during the fixation process.

One of the most used is 2% glutaraldehyde in phosphate or in cacodylate buffer solution. After this fixation, samples are fixed again in an osmium tetroxide solution at 1% buffered solution. Before this second fixation, and given the slow penetration rate of both fixatives, the samples need to be cut or "carved" creating 1 cubic millimeter in order to promote their correct fixation and to facilitate cutting and handling of the samples, in addition to the posterior observation under the microscope. After the second fixation, the third one should be with uranyl acetate as the fixative agent. The third fixation can be skipped depending on the specific needs of the sample.

II. Embedding

After the fixation of the tissue, and for its posterior observation and study in the microscope, the embedding process must start. The objective of embedding is to provide the sample with a determined consistency or hardness so as to allow for later obtaining sections or cuts of the tissue. This will also prevent fragmentation and will preserve the structure and characteristics of cells with very little interference. As far as possible, such cuts, should be fine, regular and homogeneous.

The consistency and hardness needed for the tissue is obtained by infiltrating liquid substances into the tissue. They will subsequently solidify due to refrigeration or polymerization, and the desired hardness will be obtained. Based on the sample type, and bearing in mind the technique selected for the posterior study, we can choose from among the embedding media types. According to the characteristics of embedding media, they can be classified into:

- *Hydrophilic* embedding media: such as gelatin, polyethylene glycol, and OCT.
- *Hydrophobic* embedding media: such as paraffin, celoidine, and different types of resins (such as acrylic, polyester, or epoxy resins).

Tissue Embedding in Hydrophilic Embedding Media

Bearing in mind that tissues are mainly composed of water, and that hydrophilic embedding media are soluble in water, this type of embedding allows us to work directly with the hydrated tissue. Within this embedding type, we find, among others:

Gelatin

If the tissue has previously been fixed, before starting gelatin embedding, such fixture has to be removed from the tissue through washes in running water. Since gelatin is water soluble, there is no need to dehydrate or rinse the tissue. Another advantage of gelatin is that its melting point is low. Therefore, tissue samples are spared the downsides of working with high temperatures (>40ºC) during the process. Embedding takes place by means of successive baths in gelatin with different increasing concentrations at 37ºC.

OCT (Optimal Cutting Temperature Compound)

The OCT is composed of polyvinyl alcohol, polyethylene glycol, and reserved composition excipients (Ames type) acting as cryoprotectants.

This type of embedding is currently the most widely used for obtaining frozen cuts, because it favors cutting in cryostats at very low temperatures (-20ºC) and, therefore, allows us to work with samples with no need for previous fixation.

Tissue Embedding in Hydrophobic Embedding Media

These embedding media, since they are not water miscible, force us to perform a series of previous steps to the embedding media in order to remove all the water that the tissue contains. If the sample is not correctly embedded in the embedding medium, it will spoil, and performing regular and homogeneous cuts will be very difficult. Among hydrophobic embedding media, paraffin is currently the most often used. We also find celoidine, but less frequently. There are other embedding hydrophobic media, such as different types of resins (acrylic, polyester, epoxy), that are chosen based on the type of technique subsequently used and the type of microscopy used for the visualization. Since paraffin is the most common embedding medium, we will focus on it, and will use paraffin to explain the different steps needed and in common, with certain differences for all embeddings with hydrophobic embedding media.

Paraffin Embedding

Paraffin is formed by mixtures of saturated hydrocarbons. It is solid at room temperature, and depending on its type of hydrocarbon mixture, has a melting point ranging from 40ºC to 70ºC. The most used paraffins normally have a melting point around 60ºC.

Paraffin is not water miscible. And taking into account that most fixatives, and tissues themselves, contain water, we have to take a series of steps to replace that water with an organic solvent to allow the liquid paraffin to correctly embed the tissue. We divide those steps into:

1. *Dehydration.* Dehydration is the process by which water is completely removed from the sample to be embedded. It takes place by means of chemical agents or dehydration reactants, or through physicochemical procedures (cryodesiccation and cryosubstitution). The dehydration process takes place through repeated baths in increasing alcohol content solutions (50º, 70º, 80º, 96º, 100º (absolute alcohol)). It is performed gradually so as to prevent the tissue from retracting. According to the type of tissue and sample size, the optimal time and number of baths in different concentrations is calculated to avoid a too long exposition that could cause an excessive tissue hardening. The main dehydration agents are: ethyl alcohol (the most used), methyl alcohol, acetone, butyl alcohol, dioxane, isopropyl alcohol, etc. The main characteristics of a good dehydration agent are: it must not alter tissue structures and must be miscible with the intermediate solvent or the clearing agent that will be subsequently used.
2. *Clearing or dealcoholisation.* This is the process through which the dehydration agent is substituted by a substance miscible with the embedding medium that will be used. The clearing process takes place by means of successive baths in the chosen clearing agent. The duration and amount of these baths depends on the characteristics of

the clearing liquid and the type and size of the tissue sample. The selection of the clearing agent or the intermediate solvent will be mainly based on its own characteristics, including: speed for the removal of the dehydration agent, lack of hardening or tissue retraction, appropriateness to the dehydration agent and the embedding medium, etc. The main clearing agents or intermediate solvents are: xylene, toluene, chloroform.

3. *Infiltration or Impregnation.* This is the process through which we fully infiltrate or fill the tissue sample with the chosen embedding medium. The objective of this process is to completely occupy with inclusion medium the space that was previously occupied with the water contained in the tissue. This way, we provide the homogeneity and hardness necessary for obtaining fine quality cuts of the study sample. The infiltration or impregnation process takes place through successive baths in liquid paraffin. These baths must be changed frequently, since they get saturated with clearing agent and this could generate changes in paraffin characteristics, thus hampering the posterior trimming. The length and number of baths in liquid paraffin will depend, as always, on the characteristics of the chosen paraffin (and the inclusion medium of use at that moment), as well as the type and size of the tissue sample.

   Currently, there are automatic processors, which have different vases or recipients to perform the baths in the different liquids and thermal vases for paraffins with a mechanic transport system across them that is regulated by a time programmer. This enables performing the embedding process on a high number of samples and optimizes time, since the process can continue over night.

4. *Block Preparation.* This is the process through which we obtain a tissue block embedded in the embedding medium through slow cooling until reaching 10ºC-15ºC. In order to facilitate sample identification, the embedding process and the posterior block preparation, the sample is placed in a kind of capsule or cassette. These cassettes allow for maintaining the sample immersed in a

liquid by means of the opening for infiltration they have on their entire surface.

Apart from cassettes, for block preparation, we need special molds. These molds are normally metallic (favors cooling) and of different sizes than can be adjusted to the sample size. These molds fit perfectly in the cassettes used for embedding. In summary, cassettes facilitate block preparation, their arrangement in the microtome for the obtaining of tissue sections or cuts, and their subsequent archiving.

In order to create the blocks, certain devices called "embedding stations" will be used. These stations have a liquid paraffin dispenser, a hot plate with light and a magnifier for sample orientation, and a cold plate for solidification of the block.

Tissue Embedding in Other Hydrophobic Embedding Media

Embedding media other than paraffin are normally chosen when the tissue characteristics so require such as when a tissue is too hard (undecalcified bones), when it contains structures that become affected by heat (enzyme study), when the tissue has several parts with different consistencies, or when the study requires very thick or very thin cuts. Among these other hydrophobic embedding media, plastic embedding stands out.

Plastic Embedding

This type of embedding uses acrylic resins (methylmethacrylate, glycol methacrylate, etc.) or epoxi type, and is based on the polymerization of an elemental substance of low molecular weight until transforming it into a solid, clear, and very hard compound. The following stand out:

- *Methylmethacrylate Embedding.* The elemental substance used here as an embedding medium is monomeric methylmethacrylate. This type of embedding is chosen for very hard tissue samples, such as undecalcified bones. One advantage of methacrylates is that their elasticity and hardness can be modified according to the amount of monomers that the final mixture contains. This allows for adapting to the tissue type to be embedded.

- *Embedding for Electron Microscopy.* To observe the cell's ultrastructure, it is indispensable to obtain very thin tissue cuts (nanomers), called ultrathin cuts, and to use a transmission electron microscope. In order to obtain ultrathin cuts, the tissue needs to be hardened. To that end, the most used media to embed tissue are the epoxi-type resins, or, less frequently, acrylic resins (methacrylate). In electron microscopy, the embedding process is very similar to paraffin embedding, since the same steps have to be followed, but with different substances: fixation (glutaraldehyde), post-fixation, dehydration (ethanol and acetone), intermediate solvents (epoxypropane or propylene oxide), embedding and polymerization in the embedding medium (60ºC) (epoxy resins: araldite, Epon resin, Spurr's resin).

III. Obtention of Tissue Cuts

In order to observe the characteristics of the different tissues and their cell structures through various microscopes, very thin cuts need to be performed. Otherwise, problems with light diffusion and penetration appear in optical microscopes, and electron penetration in transmission electron microscopes. The ideal thickness of cuts for their correct observation ranges from a few nanomers to hundreds of microns. The thinner the tissue sample cut has to be, the harder the tissue needs to be. Its hardness will depend on the tissue characteristics, the fixation process, the embedding process, and the selection of the embedding medium. Another way of hardening the tissue is through freezing.

In order to obtain such cuts of tissue samples, some devices called microtomes are used. These devices allow for performing cuts of micrometric thickness, fine enough to be observed with microscopes. There are different types of microtomes, such as: oscillating or rocking microtome, Minot-type or rotary microtome, sliding microtome, freezing microtome, cryostat, cryomicrotome, and ultramicrotome. The selection of the microtome type will depend on the desired thickness of the cuts, the embedding medium where the tissue is immersed, and the tissue hardening process, which can be by freezing or embedding. Microtomes for tissues embedded in paraffin are the most commonly used for optical microscopy, and ultramicrotome for transmission electron microscopy. Cryostat is also frequently used for optical microscopy, since it allows for sectioning unembedded tissue, and even tissue without fixation, resulting in a time saving and an easier process.

IV. Staining

Once our sample is cut, the next issue to address is the fact that human and animal tissues normally are colorless. Exceptions include certain parts where melanic pigments can be found in cells, colored erythrocytes, or some type of metallic deposits, or other materials coloring cell cytoplasms. Since sample structures are not apparent without staining, they need to undergo that process. To do so, we exploit the capacity of tissues to incorporate and fix colored substances in their interior.

These substances, which we call dyes, normally derive from benzene, which is an aromatic hydrocarbon with a characteristic ring in its molecular structure. These substances can have a natural origin, either plants or animals, or can derive from aniline, which is artificially obtained from tar or coal.

These dyes are classified according to their *staining affinity* for the various components of tissues. Thus, there are *alkaline dyes*, which are aniline molecules containing one or more positive charges in the molecule's colored portion. They have affinity for the acid structures of the tissue, such as nucleic acids, and nuclear structures, such as hematoxylin. *Acid dyes* are anilines that include negative charge in the molecule's colored portion. They show affinity for basic structures in cells and tissues, such as cell cytoplasm. Eoisin is an example. There are also *neutral dyes* using another type of system, such as physical impregnation, to stain tissues.

Tissue components that react with alkaline dyes are called *Basophilic dyes*, whereas components or structures reacting with acid dyes are called *Acidophilic dyes*.

Also available are other dyes called metachromatic dyes, which show *Metachromasia* when staining. They include toluidine blue and thionine. Metachromasia is the property by which, when dyes get fixed to determined tissue structures, these structures become stained in a different color other than their own. This happens because the staining molecule polymerizes when it comes into contact with certain polyanion-rich tissue parts. The resulting polymer has light absorption properties different from those of the original molecule. These cell or tissue structures that are dyed differently with metachromatic dyes are called chromatropes. For example, if toluidine blue was used as metachromatic dye, the result would be a tissue mostly dyed blue, and certain structures such as mast cell granules, or the fundamental matter of cartilages could be purple dyed.

Dyes have different *means of action* when it comes to fixing into tissues. The means may be *physical* in which the solvent acts as a mode of transport for the dye molecules that are more soluble in the tissue than in the solvent. This is normally the most characteristic course of action in fat staining. Another case is based on great volume dye molecules selectively depositing, forming insoluble molecular aggregates on certain structures, and becoming trapped in the tissue, within the net of fibers and cells. This is the case of silver impregnation.

Chemical methods are based on the appearance of a chemical reaction between the structure which is the object of the staining, and the dye itself, resulting in a new chromogen. These methods are unique to histochemistry.

Physicochemical mechanisms are based on unions between molecules due to their electrostatic charge. Molecules with different charges unite. Stainings where acid structures join alkaline dyes, and alkaline structures join acid dyes are based on this mechanism, as it has previously been discussed for basophilia and acidophilia.

Generally, when we dyed our samples, we found that the vast majority of dyes are water-soluble. The cut obtained from the paraffin block is embedded in this substance, which is not water miscible. Thus, in order to stain the samples, they need to undergo a process in which all the paraffin is removed from the cuts, and the tissue is then left in an aqueous medium. Such process is called *Deparaffinization*. It is the antagonistic process to the one suffered by the sample when it was embedded in paraffin. It basically includes the same elements but in the opposite order. Therefore, the samples will first be subject to successive baths in xylene, which will remove all paraffin from the tissue. The samples can be introduced for a few minutes in a heater at 60ºC to help in this process, as this will turn the paraffin into a liquid state, and it will be more easily removed. After that, the sample will be bathed several times in absolute ethanol, to take the xylene away completely. Afterwards, the sample will be bathed again several times in ethanol 96% in order to hydrate the sample little by little. Then, the sample will repeatedly be bathed in running water. Some laboratories add more ethanol steps with decreasing concentrations before starting with water. But these two steps cited above are the strictly necessary ones, except in the case of an especially delicate sample.

Once our sample is stained, and before placing it under the microscope, the sample needs to undergo the *mounting process*. This process involves preparing the sample to be as clearly observable as possible under the microscope. And, at the same time, gives us the option to preserve the already stained sample for aftertime and successive observations. The easiest way to do that is by placing a coverslip on the sample. This is used for *in vivo* samples stained with vital dyes. These samples are not expected to last for a long time; they are prepared for a particular observation. Some stainings or techniques need mounting in an aqueous medium, because a different mounting would interfere with the staining, creating artefacts or impeding their observation. This is the case of fluorescence, and sometimes certain immunohistochemical products. In those cases, the sample is covered with a mounting medium such as gelatin or buffered glycerin, and a coverslip is placed on it. It is then sealed with lacquer to increase its durability. Even then, this type of sample has a very limited duration, since it is easily degraded. The *permanent mounting* of samples takes place in a resin medium, which apart from preserving, also improves the light refractive index, thus helping to achieve a better observation under the optical microscope. Nowadays, the most common method is to use artificial resins. But in the past, resins from trees such as Canada balsam or Dammar gum were normally used. These resins are not water miscible. Therefore, again, the sample will have to undergo a process in which water will be replaced with ethanol in an increasing concentration. And that ethanol will be followed by baths in xylene to remove the ethanol from the tissue, and prepare the sample for the resin. These baths in xylene are also called rinse. And once the xylene and ethanol are both totally removed, some drops of resin or mounting medium will be put on the sample, and a coverslip will be placed on it, preventing the formation of bubbles as far as practicable. When the resin is dry, the sample is then ready for observation under the microscope. And its durability is quite long.

Next, we proceed to describe some of the techniques most frequently used for studying liver biopsies.

Hematoxylin-Eoisin Technique

This is one of the most used techniques in laboratory practice, both for clinical diagnosis and research. This technique is very adequate for a general vision of the tissue, which will show distinguishably nuclear staining, and cytoplasm staining. It is very simple, consists of only two steps, and is quick. Nuclear staining takes place through hematoxylin staining, cytoplasm staining, and the background eosin staining. Staining in these two dyes is based on physicochemical methods. Therefore, to sum up, hematoxylin is basophilic and will stain acid structures in the tissue; eosin is acidophilic and will complement the process by staining alkaline structures in the tissue.

In the particular case of a *liver biopsy*, this technique is useful to assess the grade of preservation of liver structures, to detect Mallory bodies, and to assess cell ballooning.

The first part of the staining is made with hematoxylin, which is a vegetal origin dye extracted from logwood trees (*Haematoxylum Campechianum*) originating from Central America. A substance is extracted in the form of crystals that turn purple when they oxidize. This substance is used as a dye in the textile industry. These crystals have no staining capacities. They need to undergo an oxidation process to obtain a substance called hematein. This oxidation process can take place spontaneously when the crystals are exposed to atmospheric oxygen, or be induced by adding oxidizing chemical agents. Apart from these oxidizing agents, metallic salts are usually added, and they provide a greater staining capacity and a more specific affinity for acid structures, which are stained in the blue range of colors. Depending on the type of metallic salt used, different types of hematoxylin will be obtained: aluminum hematoxylin such as Harris' or Mayer's, iron hematoxylins such as Weigert's or Hedenhaim's, chrome hematoxylin, etc. each with its pros and cons. In our case, we used Carazzi's hematoxylin, since we have been very pleased with the results.

The second part of the staining is performed by Eosin, which is a xanthene dye obtained from the interaction of bromine with fluorescein, which contributes with its characteristic autofluorescence. As a result, there are two types of eosin: yellowish or eosin Y, and bluish or eosin B that differ according to the bromine atoms they contain. Eosin Y has a greater content, and is the one we chose to use. It shows staining affinity for cell and tissue alkaline structures, staining them in colors ranging from orangey to pink or red. It can be used both in water and alcohol solutions. In water solutions, it is necessary to add some type of substance protecting it from contamination, such as thymol or formol drops.

The reagents needed for this technique are:

Carazzi's Hematoxylin:

- 1 gram hematoxylin
- 0.2 grams potassium iodate
- 50 grams potassium alum
- 200 milliliters glycerin
- 800 milliliters distilled water

  The reagents are added, in order, to a mortar in which they homogenize before the next reagent is added. In the end, a fine powder is obtained, which will then be slowly mixed with glycerin. Finally, water will be added, and the resulting mixture will be left for oxidation in contact with light and atmospheric oxygen for 15 days before use.

Watery Eosin:

- 5 grams yellowish eosin or eosin Y
- 500 milliliters distilled water

Some thymol will be added to the eosin solution in order to prevent its contamination.

The *technical procedure* is as follows:

- Dewax and hydrate the cuts.
- Introduce the cuts in Carazzi's hematoxylin, from 10 to 15 minutes, depending on its maturation or oxidation state.
- Wash off in running water for 10 minutes, until the purple color of the cuts turns blue.
- Introduce the cuts in eosin for 30 seconds.
- Without washing, dehydrate, clear and mount with resin.

During dehydration of the samples, eosin also differentiates, thus removing its excess.

Results will show nuclei and nucleic acids in a range of blues, cytoplasm in orangey or pinkish, and cell structures such as collagen in pink. This way, staining will be useful for observing the general structure and the cell state of our liver biopsy.

Masson's Technique

Masson's technique is a trichrome stain designed for observing collagen fibers and connective tissue. In trichrome staining, dyes are normally intended for differentially staining various tissue structures. Thus, a nuclear stain, a cytoplasmic stain, and a collagen fiber stain will be used. Differential staining is founded, in part, upon the size of pores in various tissue components when the proteins reticulate as a result of fixation, which is much laxer in collagen structures than in cell cytoplasm structures. And it also partly depends on the treatment with phosphotungstic acid and phosphomolybdic acid underwent by the tissue to improve the affinity of collagen fibers for the dye.

This technique is of special interest in the case of liver biopsy for observing and assessing the degree of distribution of fibrosis.

If the samples have been fixed in formol, treatment with Bouin's fixative solution is appropriate, since it will act as mordant for the next staining.

The *reagents* that used are:

Weigert's Iron Hematoxylin

Solution A

- 1 gr hematoxylin
- 100 mL absolute ethanol

Solution B

- 4 mL ferric chloride at 29%
- 95 mL distilled water
- 1 mL hydrochloric acid

At the time of use, a working solution is generated by mixing solution A and B in equal proportions and well mixed.

Biebrich Scarlet and Acid Fucsin Solution

- 90 mL of Biebrich Scarlet in aqueous solution at 1%
- 10 mL of Acid Fucsin in aqueous solution at 1%
- 1 mL glacial acetic acid

Phosphotungstic Acid and Phosphomolybdic Acid Solution

- 5 gr phosphotungstic acid
- 5 gr phosphomolybdic acid
- 200 mL distilled water

Aniline Blue Solution

- 2.5 gr aniline blue
- 2 mL glacial acetic acid
- 100 mL distilled water

Acetic Acid Solution at 1%

- 1 mL glacial acetic acid
- 99 mL distilled water

The *technical procedure* is as follows:

- Dewax and hydrate the cuts.

- Wash off in distilled water.
- If the fixation has not been carried out with Bouin's fixative, perform a post-fixation with Bouin's solution for 12 hours at room temperature, or for one hour in a heater at 58-60ºC.
- Wash off with abundant running water to remove all fixative remaining. Then wash off in distilled water.
- Dye with Weigert iron hematoxylin for 10 minutes.
- Wash off in running water for 10 minutes.
- Wash off with distilled water.
- Dye with the Biebrich Scarlet and Acid Fucsin solution for 15 minutes.
- Wash off with distilled water.
- Differentiate the cuts with the phosphotungstic-phosphomolybdic acid solution from 10 to 15 minutes.
- Dye with aniline blue from 5 to 10 minutes.
- Differentiate the cuts with the acetic acid solution at 1% from 2 to 3 minutes.
- Wash off in distilled water.

During the staining, we can control microscopically whether or not the phosphotungstic-phosphomolybdic acid solution has correctly differentiated and that the collagen fibers of the tissue do not appear red. If, after differentiation, the red color persisted, that means that the acid solution needs more time to act.

The *results* will show the nucleus dyed in black, muscle fibers, cytoplams and keratin in red tones, and collagen fibers in deep blue.

Gomori's Reticulin Technique

This is a silver impregnation technique. This type of technique relies on silver salts that react with certain parts of tissues, normally electronegative structures that can attract silver ions. These ions, once fixed onto the structures, are forced to precipitate by means of the action of reducing agents, delivering a metallic silver pigment. Gomori's technique, more precisely, is a two-stage silver impregnation that uses potassium hydroxide as the source and formol as the reducing agent. It uses potassium permanganate as oxidizing agent, potassium disulphite to whiten the cuts, and ferric alum as mordent.

The optimal result for this method depends in part on the wash that takes place before reduction with formol. Its duration should be determined empirically. It is also important to tone the samples with gold chloride. This gives a bluish grey color to precipitated silver, removes unspecific silver remnants, and gives collagen fibers a purple color.

With this technique in *liver biopsies*, as in previous cases, we observe and assess the distribution degree of fibrosis.

Neutral formol at 10% is recommended as the most adequate fixation. This technique can be used in paraffin, celoidine and freezing cuts. Cuts are recommended to be 6-7 microns thick, so as to allow for following the course of reticular fibers in tissue thickness.

The *reagents* that will be used are:

Potassium Disulphite at 2%

- 4 gr potassium disulphite
- 200 mL distilled water

Ferric Alum at 2%

- 4 gr ferric alum
- 200 mL distilled water

Ammoniacal Silver Solution

- 25 mL silver nitrate at 10%
- 5 mL sodium hydroxide at 10%

These two solutions are mixed, and ammonia is added drop by drop, until the silver precipitate is completely dissolved, and the resulting solution is completely transparent. To the consequential solution volume, an equivalent volume of distilled water is added. It is then filtered and let set for 12 hours in the dark. The excess of ammonia will evaporate. Once evaporated, this solution is preserved in a refrigerator at 4°C and protected from light.

Neutral Formol at 10%

- 20 mL commercial formalin
- 180 mL distilled water

The solution's pH is measured and then adjusted to pH 7, using a sodium hydroxide solution.

Gold Chloride at 0.2%

- 0.4 gr gold chloride
- 200 mL distilled water

Sodium Thiosulphate at 2.5%

- 5 gr sodium thiosulphate
- 200 mL distilled water

Neutral Red at 1%

- 2 gr neutral red
- 200 mL distilled water

The *technical procedure* is:

- Dewax and hydrate the cuts.
- Wash off with distilled water.
- Cover the cuts with potassium permanganate at 1% for 2 minutes.
- Wash off in distilled water.
- Whiten the cuts with potassium disulphite solution at 2% for 1 minute.
- Wash off thoroughly in distilled water several times.
- Treat the cuts with ferric alum at 2% for 1 minute.
- Wash off twice with distilled water.
- Treat the cuts with previously filtered ammoniacal silver solution for 1 minute.
- Wash off the cuts in distilled water for 5 minutes making several changes.
- Reduce the cuts with neutral formol at 10% for 5 minutes.

- Wash off thoroughly with distilled water.
- Treat the cuts with gold chloride solution at 0.2% from 5 to 10 minutes.
- Wash off in distilled water.
- Add potassium disulphite at 2% for 1 minute.
- Wash off in distilled water.
- Treat the cuts with sodium thiosulphate at 2.5% from 1 to 2 minutes.
- Wash off with distilled water.
- Optionally, stain once with neutral red at 1% as a nuclear stain acting as a contrast.
- Wash off with distilled water.
- Dehydrate, clear and mount in resin.

The *results* will show reticular fibers in black, nucleus in grey, and collagen in a light purple tone. If the sample has been contrasted with neutral red, then cell nucleus will appear black.

PAS Technique

This technique's name is an acronym for Periodic Acid Schiff, which is the main reagent in this histochemical technique. This technique is much used for determining mucopolysaccharides, glycoproteins, glycolipids, simple polysaccharides... Schiff reagent is obtained by modifying basic fucsin treating it with sulphurous acid, thus making it lose its characteristic fuchsia color and turning it colorless. Then, when it reacts with carbonyl groups in the tissues, it retrieves its broken double bond and regains its fuchsia color.

Before using Schiff reagent, the technique requires that the tissue has previously been oxydated using periodic acid. This increases the amount of carbonyl groups present in carbohydrates, to make them more evident.

Nuclear staining is generally used as contrast with hematoxylin. In our case, we will use Carazzi's hematoxylin.

In the particular case of liver biopsy, this technique is useful for observing cell glycogen content, and assessing the degree of metabolic alteration suffered by hepatocytes. Hepatocyte content can also be observed in lipofucsin pigment, which is a brown color pigment that appears in cell cytoplasm as a consequence of fatty acids degradation, and affects cell functionality.

The *reagents* that will be used are:

Carazzi's Hematoxylin

Periodic Acid at 2.5%

- 5 gr periodic acid
- 200 mL distilled water

Shiff Reagent

- 0.25 gr basic diamond fucsin in crystals
- 6 gr sodium dithionite
- 300 mL distilled water

To elaborate, fucsin is blended in a mortar and 150 mL distilled water is added. Separately, the sodium dithionite is mixed with the other 150 mL of distilled water. These are individually filtered, and then slowly mixed by pouring the sodium dithionite solution into the basic fucsin one. The result will be a clear and opalescent solution that must be preserved in a refrigerator at 4ºC and protected from light.

Sodium Disulphite at 2%

- 4 gr sodium disulphite
- 200 mL distilled water

The *technical procedure* is as follows:

- Dewax and hydrate the cuts.
- Treat the cuts with periodic acid at 2.5% for 10 minutes.
- Wash off in running water for 10 minutes.
- Wash off in distilled water.
- Dye the cuts with Schiff reagent for 15 minutes, preferably protected from light.

- Treat with sodium dishulphite at 2% from 3 to 5 minutes.
- Wash off in running water for 10 minutes.
- Wash off in distilled water.
- Dye the cuts with Carazzi's hematoxylin for 5 minutes.
- Wash off the cuts in running water for 10 minutes.
- Dehydrate, clear and mount with resin.

The *results* will show the nucleus in blue, and the positive PAS material in the range of pink to fuchsia. Glycolypids, gangliosides and cerebrosides, mucoproteins in general, neutral mucopolysaccharides, simple polysaccharides like glycogen or glycoproteins of the basal membrane, are all considered to be PAS positive substances. The lipofuscin pigment is also PAS positive.

Perls' Prussian Blue Technique

This is a technique destined for the detection of free iron ions in the tissue, as well as their deposits, such as hemosiderin. Hemosiderin is the deposits of ferric hydroxide that appear in cell cytoplasm or inside macrophages. They are usually the result of natural or pathological degradation of hemoglobin.

The *reagents* that will be used are:

Potassium Ferrocyanide at 5%

- 10 gr potassium ferrocyanide
- 200 mL distilled water

Hydrochloric acid at 5%

- 10 mL commercial hydrochloric acid
- 190 mL distilled water

Carazzi's Hematoxylin

The *technical procedure* is as follows:

- Dewax and hydrate the cuts.

- Wash off with running water.
- Treat the cuts with a potassium ferrocyanide solution at 5% and hydrochloric acid at 5%, equal proportions, for 20 minutes.
- Wash off thoroughly with running water.
- Dye the cuts with Carazzi's hematoxylin for 5 minutes.
- Wash off in running water for 10 minutes.
- Dehydrate, clear and mount with resin.

The *results* will show iron granules in light blue, the cell nucleus in dark blue, and cytoplasms in yellow.

Specific Techniques for Fats

When working to detect fats, their physicochemical properties must be taken into account, because they will limit the methodologies to be used with them in the laboratory. Lipids are water insoluble, but they are very soluble in certain organic solvents, such as ethanol, acetone, chloroform, toluene or xylene. This feature will prevent them from being embedded in paraffin, since the lipid material would get lost in the process. Therefore, embeddings can only take place in water soluble media, such as gelatin. As an alternative frozen cuts of previously embedded material can be used.

The most appropriate fixative for the lipid material is formol, because of its good results when fixing neutral fats. If calcium chloride is also added to it, results are even more improved. This is because calcium ions will make lipids be more stable, and formol will then be able to fix them more efficiently.

When dying, the technique will highlight the presence of homophasic lipid tissue, which is the one to be found in very specific locations in the cell, such as the cytoplasm, without being mixed with any other element. Heterophasic lipids are dispersed throughout the cell territory, and they are mixed with other substances. It is very difficult to determine their presence.

The staining mechanism to detect these homophasic lipids is a purely physical mechanism, which has much to do with the solubility characteristics of lipids. It is based on the fact that the dye is better dissolved in the lipid than in the medium that will be used for the technique (it will normally be ethanol or acetone). Consequently, there is a trend for dye molecules to migrate from the solution used into tissue lipids. The longer the sample is exposed to the solution with dye, the more intense the resulting color will be. This is because molecules accumulate gradually in lipid deposits.

As a general rule, the solutions of these dyes specific for fats are not usually very stable. Therefore, when possible, it is recommended to make them at the time of use. When that is not possible, the best option is to store them in an airtight container, because instability could make the dye precipitate and then deliver false positives.

When we made these techniques, we selected the cryostat cut of tissue already fixed. We made cuts of 7 to 10 microns. The next explanations of procedures that follow will be made bearing in mind cuts of these characteristics. It also has to be taken into account that since these preparations are made with aqueous mounting, their life is very limited- no more than 15 days it they are conserved at 4°C in a refrigerator.

Sudan IV Technique

This dye is specific for neutral fats. Special care will be required, since the dye precipitates very easily. Carazzi's hematoxylin will be used as a nuclear contrast dye, since in the Sudan IV technique there are only the lipids of the tissue, and contrast dye is very convenient to put them in context. This hematoxylin can be replaced by any other hematoxylin or by other nuclear dyes.

The *reagents* that will be used are:

Sudan IV Solution

- 1 gr Sudan IV solution
- 50 mL acetone
- 50 mL ethanol at 70%

The *technical procedure* is:

- Wash off cuts in ethanol at 70%.
- Treat the cuts with the Sudan IV solution for 10 minutes.
- Wash off with ethanol at 70%.

- Wash off in distilled water.
- Dye with Carazzi's hematoxylin for 5 minutes.
- Wash off in running water for 10 minutes.
- Without dehydrating, mount in an aqueous medium and seal with a lacquer.

The *results* will show the nucleus in blue, and lipids in a range from orangey-reddish to intense red.

Sudan Black Technique

This dye, as its name indicates, is black. Therefore, we recommend contrast dye for the nucleus with some dye such as neutral red, in order to help acquire a better general picture.

The *reagents* that will be used are:

Sudan Black Solution

- 1 gr Black Sudan solution
- 50 mL acetone
- 50 mL ethanol at 70%

The *technical procedure* is:

- Wash off cuts in ethanol at 70%.
- Treat the cuts with the Sudan Black solution for 10 minutes.
- Wash off with ethanol at 70%.
- Wash off in distilled water.
- Dye with neutral red for 2 minutes.
- Wash off in running water for 10 minutes.
- Without dehydrating, mount in an aqueous medium and seal with a lacquer.

The *results* will show lipids and myelin in black; and if a contrast dye has been performed with neutral red, the nucleus will appear in red.

Sudan Red or III Technique

This technique can also be used in paraffin cuts, bearing in mind that after the embedding process, the amount of lipids that will appear will be much lower than that of the tissue before the embedding process.

The *reagents* that will be used are:

Carazzi's Hematoxylin

Sudan III Solution

- 2 gr Sudan III solution
- 100 mL ethanol at 70%
- 100 mL acetone
- 2 gr Scarlet red

First, Sudan III solution is dissolved into the ethanol at 70%. Once it has been dissolved, acetone is added. And when it is homogeneous, it is dissolved again in Scarlet red. It is very important to thoroughly filtrate this solution before it is applied to the sample so as to prevent the formation of precipitates that could lead to false positives.

The *technical procedure* is:

- Dewax cuts and rehydrate with ethanol 96º.
- Wash off the cuts with ethanol at 50% for 1 minute.
- Treat the cuts with the Sudan III solution that has been previously filtered for 15 minutes in a heater at 60ºC, or for 1 hour at room temperature.
- Quickly wash off the cuts in ethanol at 50%.
- Quickly wash off in distilled water.
- Dye the cuts with Carazzi's hematoxylin for 5 minutes.
- Wash off in water for 10 minutes.
- Mount it in an aqueous medium and seal with a lacquer.

The *results* will show the nucleus in blue, and lipids dyed in red or orangey red.

Oil Red-O Technique

This technique can also be applied to paraffin cuts, bearing in mind that, as in the last case, most of the fats will get lost in the embedding process.

The *reagents* that will be used are:

Propylene glycol at 85%

- 85 mL commercial propylene glycol
- 15 mL distilled water

Carazzi's Hematoxylin

Oil Red-O Solution at 0.5%

- 0.5 gr Oil Red-O
- 100 mL commercial propylene glycol

To prepare Oil Red-O, it is placed in a mortar and a small amount of propylene glycol is added. Then it must be blended and the sample homogenized by gradually adding the rest of propylene glycol. After that, the solution is heated to 95ºC, while continuously stirred until the rest of stain is dissolved. Once it is hot, it is filtered with filter paper and left to rest all night through. The next morning, it will be filtered again through a glass-fiber filter with the help of a vacuum system. If the resulting solution is cloudy, a new filtration must be performed.

The *technical procedure* is:

- Dewax and hydrate the cuts.
- Wash off with propylene glycol at 100% for 5 minutes.
- Dye with the Oil Red-O solution from 48 to 72 hours.
- Wash off the cuts with propylene glycol at 85% from 1 to 2 minutes.
- Dye the cuts with Carazzi's hematoxylin for 5 minutes.
- Wash off in running water for 10 minutes.
- Wash off several times with distilled water.
- Mount it in an aqueous medium and seal with a lacquer.

The *results* will show lipids in red color, and the nucleus in blue tones.

IMMUNOHISTOCHEMICAL TECHNIQUES

Immunohistochemistry is a process through which a specific antigen can be detected, amplified and visualized both at tissue and cell levels. This is achieved by means of the antigen-antibody reaction, which is very specific and of high affinity. In immunohistochemistry, selected antibodies are used to identify specific antigens. In immunohistochemistry, antigen is any substance or molecule that we want to detect. In order to visualize the site where the antigen-antibody reaction takes place, a tracker or marker is needed. Such marking can be done with fluorochromes (immunofluorescence techniques), with enzymes (immunoenzymatic techniques), with metallic ions in colloidal form (immuno-oro technique) or with radioactive isotopes. The antigen can be detected both through direct marking of the primary antibody (direct method), or indirectly using a secondary or even a tertiary antibody.

In order to better understand the technique and the antigen-antibody reaction, we will explain some basic concepts:

- *Immune response.* This response lays in the identification of a foreign agent. Such identification takes place through two types of molecules: T-cell receptors and immunoglobulines.
- *Antigen.* The substance or substances capable of producing an immune response, either humoral or cellular, or both at the same time (immunogenicity), capable of combining with antibodies and with cell receptors (antigenicity), and capable of producing an allergic reaction (allergenicity). Each antibody is specific for a determined antigen, and binds to a determined part of it, called epitome or antigenic determinant, thus establishing the antigen-antibody specificity.
- *Antibody.* The molecules with antibody activity are generically designated as immunoglobulins. All immunoglobulin molecules

present a common structure composed of four polypeptide chains, two long chains (H or heavy chains) and two short chains (L or light chains). According to the primary structure of their heavy chains, they are divided into five classes, and are termed Ig G, Ig A, Ig M, Ig D, and Ig E.

Immunohistochemical Detection Systems

Direct Method

This is the simplest method, and involves only one step applying the specific antibody against the antigen that one wants to demonstrate. The antibody is conjugated with a marker (either fluorescent or enzymatic) that makes the reaction visible under the microscope.

Indirect Method

The first antibody is specific for the antigen that we want to demonstrate, and it is not conjugated with any marker. A second antibody has to be used (developed in an animal of a different species from the first). This second antibody can be marked or not (the second antibody is specific for the first antibody). If the second antibody is not marked, a third antibody (developed in the same animal species as the first) is used. This third antibody is marked.

Types of Immunohistochemical Techniques

Based on the marker (fluorochrome, enzymes, etc.) and the detection system used (direct or indirect method), different types of immunohistochemical techniques can be found.

Immunofluorescence Techniques

Fluorescence is a form of luminescence, understood as the emission of light generated by a non-thermal energy source, and under the effect of an excitation. Primary fluorescence (autofluorescence) is that spontaneously presented by certain substances. In tissues that do not have this property, fluorescence can be induced (secondary fluorescence) through immunohistochemical techniques, using fluorescent molecules, named fluorochromes, as markers. Fluorochromes are chemical molecules that absorb light at a certain wavelength and deliver a different one. Their excitation spectrums and emissions vary according to the fluorochrome used. The most used fluorochromes in immunofluorescence techniques are: fluorescein, rhodamine, Alexa Fluor, DyLight Fluor, etc. The disadvantage of this type of technique is that it is not permanent marking, since the light emitted by the fluorescent molecule (fluorochrome) vanishes with time. Therefore, it must be preserved from light. In order to visualize the results of this technique type, a special microscope is necessary: fluorescence microscope.

Immunoperoxidase Techniques

In this technique type, peroxidase is the marker used. Peroxidase is an enzyme obtained from horseradish, and it is the most used enzyme tracker. Peroxidase can be used both bonded to the primary antibody (direct technique, the simplest method, but less sensitive for antigens detection) and in immunocomplexes called PAP (peroxidase+antiperoxidase antibody) that will join a bridging antibody (secondary antibody) in the indirect technique. These PAP complexes will be the tracers for the antigen-antibody reaction. Next, the marker will be developed by oxygenated water (H2O2) added as substrate, together with the chromogen appropriate for that enzyme. The reaction takes place when the enzyme binds to the substrate, releasing oxygen, thus causing the chromogen oxydation and originating an insoluble brown product. Peroxidase can be endogenously found in tissues.

Techniques with Alkaline Phosphatase

When tissues are very rich in endogenous peroxidase, alkaline phosphatase is used as the tracer. Sometimes, there is endogenous phosphatase but in a few number of tissues than in normal conditions. In these cases, its endogenous activity requires no inhibition. If needed, it can be inhibited with levamisole. This enzyme is developed using Naphthol-AS-

MX phosphate as a substrate, and Fast Red TR or Fast Blue BB as chromogen.

Avidin-Biotin Technique

This type of technique uses biotinylated antibodies. Biotin is a low molecular weight vitamin presenting a high affinity for avidin. Avidin is a high molecular weight glycoprotein that can be found in egg white and in the *Streptomyces avidini* bacteria (streptavidin). An almost irreversible and very rapid interaction takes place between them. Avidin has four connection points with biotin, and can be conjugated with different markers. Its specificity and affinity are much greater. It can be developed by the DAB, if the marker used is peroxidase.

Immunohistochemistry Universal Kit

Currently, there are several universal kits containing al the reagents required in the immunostaining process. Some of them even allow for indiscriminate use with monoclonal and polyclonal antibodies, and enable their development in different colors, choosing the adequate marker and chromogen. Most of these kits use indirect detection systems based on polymers. An important advantage of this detection system is that it normally is ultrasensitive with the associated primary antibody saving.

Immunohistochemistry Techniques Processes

All immunohistochemistry techniques follow a similar process. The differences that may exist in such processes are normally caused by: the type of study sample, the type of tissue used, the fixation system used, whether the sample is embedded or frozen, the embedding media used, the primary antibody to be used, the detection system, and the selected development system. The following scheme shows a summary of the process to follow, which will be discussed later.

1. Deparaffination and hydration of previously identified samples.
2. Antagonist unmasking if necessary.
3. Washout.
4. Enzymatic activity blockade.
5. Washout.
6. Background staining blockade.
7. Primary antibody incubation.
8. Washout.
9. Detection system.
10. Washout.
11. Development system.
12. Washout.
13. Counterstaining.
14. Washout.
15. Dehydration and mounting.

The entire process has to be carefully performed, avoiding whenever possible, interfering or destroying the tissue and cell structure, and conserving its immunoreactivity. All variables in the process affect the outcomes of the immunohistochemistry technique used. The loss of antigenic epitope integrity depends on them.

Fixation

For this process, sample fixation is one of the most important steps. The ideal fixative in immunohistochemistry preserves the antigens' integrity, preserves tissue and cell morphology, prevents the extraction, diffusion or displacement of antigens during the fixation process, and does not interfere with the antigen-antibody reaction. There is no universal fixative. It has to be chosen from among the antagonist groups that one wants to demonstrate. The most used fixative is formaldehyde or formalin (aqueous solution of formaldehyde). It is prepared at 10% starting with commercial formol (formaldehydes at 40%), which gives the solution a final formol concentration of 4%. This fixative generates reticles, creating bonds or cross-linked bridges, and giving as a result a net in which epitopes are masked and the primary antibody is prevented from binding the antigen.

Deparaffination and Hydration of Samples

Once the cuts have been rehydrated, it is very important to prevent them from drying out, because when cuts dry in any of the technique's steps, an unspecific staining may take place. To avoid that, the immunostaining process is performed in trays or metallic containers called moist chambers. This helps the cuts remain hydrated and prevents evaporation. A PAP pen can also be used. This is a special marker that creates a fine hydrophobic layer around the cut, which helps dilutions remain exclusively in the regions of interest and maintains the cuts hydrated. It also helps saving antibody.

Antigen Unmasking (For Tissues Fixed in Formol)

Antagonist recovery is the process through which the antigen's molecular structure is restored, and immunoreactiviy is retrieved, thus providing optimal immunohistochemical results. The methods used to obtain an antagonist recovery are:

Enzyme Unmasking

Proteolytic enzymes are normally used with proteinase K, trypsin, pepsin, pronase, etc. These enzymes facilitate the tissue penetration of antibodies, eliminating the protein net that wraps antagonist determinants through the fixation process. This method will depend on: enzyme type and concentration, time and temperature of digestion, tissue type and fixation type. Therefore, the digestion time should be adjusted to each case.

Heat-Induced Unmasking (Heat-Induced Epitope Retrieval-Hier)

Most antibodies used in tissue that has been fixed with formol and embedded in paraffin, then require this method for antigen retrieval. Variables with a greater influence on HIER effectiveness include: temperature, time, tissue fixation time, nature and pH of the retrieval buffer. HIER is normally performed through incubation in a citrate buffer or EDTA, at a temperature of 97ºC-98ºC for 20 minutes. Domestic microwaves or pressure cookers are frequently used for this. But the best option, when available, is to use a scientific microwave, which, unlike previous options, allows for accurately controlling time and temperature.

Enzyme Activity Blockade

This is a method to achieve enzyme activity inhibition for the enzyme used as a marker that can be endogenously found in the tissue. The method involves the incubation of the cuts before the immunological process, applying an agent that blocks in each specific case. If the blockade is not performed, false positives could be obtained in the immunostaining.

Background Staining Blockade

Background staining can be specific or nonspecific. Specific staining can be due to the presence of the study antigen in locations different from those where it was expected to be detected, the existence of antibodies in the primary antiserum acting against different antigens than those expected to be determined, or the passive trapping of antigens, or antigen diffusion, to places where they are not normally found. The most common nonspecific staining is the non-immunological bond of the antibody with certain tissue components, due to hydrophobic and electrostatic forces. The blockade solution binds to binding sites that are not specific inside the tissue, aiming at preventing the nonspecific bonding of primary and secondary antibodies. Cuts are incubated with a protein solution, such as bovine serum albumin (BSA) or normal serum of the same animal species as the secondary antibody. With the objective of ensuring the technique's specificity, an adequate dilution of the primary antibody needs to be achieved, preventing evaporation during incubation, and making the washes be thorough.

Primary Antibody Incubation

Depending on the chosen primary antibody, the corresponding manufacturing company will provide specific indications on its dilution ranges, time and temperature for incubation, detection method, etc. These vary based on the following: type of antibody used, detection method to be used, and whether the tissue used is embedded in paraffin and fixed in formol.

There are two types of antibodies, monoclonal and polyclonal antibodies.

- *Monoclonal* antibodies can be created in mice or rabbits. They are the product of a single clone of plasma cells. Therefore, antibody molecules are all immunohistologically identical, with only one specificity and only one affinity.
- *Polyclonal* antibodies are the mixture of immunoglobulins synthesized by different plasma cell clones that react with different epitopes on the antigen for which they were created. When the optimal dilution of primary antibody has to be determined, titration is needed. Antibody titration is the higher dilution of an antibody, resulting in the maximal specific coloration with the minimal background. It is performed through serial dilutions of an antibody stock solution (1/25; 1/50; 1/100; etc.). The habitual incubation time is one hour at room temperature, 30-60 minutes at 37ºC, and 12 hours or more in a refrigerator at 4ºC.

Detection Systems

In order to make the antibody-antigen union visible under the microscope, it is necessary to use detection and coloring systems. Several types of detection systems can be found. Some of them have already been discussed here.

Development Systems

These development systems are based on the enzyme-substrate reaction. Detection systems use enzymes to transform colorless chromogens into colorful final products as a result of oxidation. This allows for their visualization under the microscope. The most used enzymes are peroxidase and alkaline phosphatase.

Counterstaining or Contrast Staining

Counterstaining is normally used to facilitate the visualization and detection of immunostained tissue areas, distinguishing them from those areas that are not stained. This contrast staining is usually carried out with hematoxylin.

Dehydration and Mounting

Dehydration is achieved through washes in alcohols of increasing concentrations to take the cuts to xylol. The mounting used can be aqueous or permanent, depending on the chromogen type used, and on whether the resulting color product is soluble or not in alcohol and in other organic solvents.

Washes

Throughout the process, several washes are required between subsequent steps. They are performed in order to remove the excess of primary antibody and of other products used during the process. Washes are normally performed with buffered solutions to which a detergent (Triton X-100, Tween 20, etc.) is added. This detergent acts to permeabilize membranes and helps antibodies penetrate adequately and reach the antigens to be detected. Several washes of short duration (5 minutes) are usually more effective than one single longer wash. Given the large number of washes required, some cuts are frequently peeled off. Therefore, using an adhesive is recommended to fix cuts to the slide, with adhesives such as egg albumin, gelatin or poly-L-lysine. It is important not to add too much adhesive, since non-specific background staining could increase.

Controls

Controls are carried out in order to check whether the immunohistochemical technique performed is specific, and verify that there are no false negatives or positives.

Negative Controls

An omission of the primary antibody or its replacement by non-immune serum or buffered solution. The same tissue as for the positive control is used. If the results are positive, this will be due to an unspecific fixation.

Positive Controls

These are performed using a tissue cut including the antigen to demonstrate. If the result is negative, the cause is a fixation defect or an error during the technique procedure.

Automated Immunostainers

Thanks to new technologies, devices that perform automatic immunostaining can be found nowadays. They allow for the introduction of slides with tissue cuts, previously tagged with barcodes for their identification using a reader, and each sample will be applied with the correct reagent. This process is very laborious due to the precision required on each of the samples, and due to the complex electronic mechanism controlled by a computer, which comprises its own thermal source for the antigenic unmasking. This involves a great progress with a reduction in errors while the technique is performed, since times, temperatures, reagent quantities, etc. are not shortened nor exceeded.

REFERENCES

Casado Martín F., Rodríguez Sanjuán J.C., Val-Bernal F., Blanco García C., Herrero Zapatero A. Anatomopathologic and morphometric study of hepatocarcinoma. *The Spanish Journal of Gastroenterology.* 1993; 84 (5):315-8. PMID: 8305258.

De Dios Soler M., Acosta Haab G. "*Immunohistochemistry Guide for Technicians*". 1st Ed. Nacional Cancer Institute. Buenos Aires (Argentina). 2018.

Garcia de Moral Raimundo. "*Laboratory of Pathological Anatomy*". 1st Ed. Madrid (Spain). Interamericana-McGraw Hill Ed. 1993.

Gil Grande L. Blind liver biopsy in current medicine. *Rev Clin Esp.* 2003; 203(5):219-20. PMID:12765566.

Martin Lacave I., Garcia Caballero T., *Atlas of Immunohistochemistry.* 1st Ed. Madrid (Spain). Diaz de Santos Editors. 2012.

Masson P.J. "Trichrome stainings and their preliminary techniques". *J Tech Met.* 1929.

Mc Manus F.J.A. and Mowry Robert W. *"Histological Techniques".* 1st. Ed Atika. Ed. 1968.

Montuenga L. Esteban -Ruiz F.J., Calvo González A. *Techniques in Histology and Cellular Biology.* 2nd Ed. Madrid (Spain). Masson Editors. 2014.

Urpegui García A.M., Morandeira García M.J., Soria Navarro J., Rivas Rodríguez P., Valencia Julve J., Fernández Larripa S., Vallés Varela H. Immunohistochemical markers of cell proliferation in laryngeal carcinoma. *Acta Otorrinolaringol Esp.* 2000. 51(4):279-87. PMID: 10984949.

In: Liver Steatosis and Bariatric Surgery ISBN: 978-1-53616-444-2
Editors: Jaime Ruiz-Tovar et al.

Chapter 6

CONVENTIONAL IMAGING TESTS FOR THE EVALUATION OF NASH

Luis Tomás Ocaña Wilhelmi, MD, PhD,
Bruno Ramos Molina, PhD
and Enrique Glückmann Maldonado, MD
Surgery Department, University of Málaga, Málaga, Spain

ABSTRACT

In the last two decades, enormous progress has been made in the evaluation of NAFLD by non-invasive images, techniques that receive more and more attention. Among these stand out (in addition to others in research that use biological markers and image): Ultrasound, Computerized Tomography, Magnetic Resonance Imaging (PDFF), Magnetic Resonance Spectroscopy, Magnetic Resonance Elastography, Transient Elastography (VCTE, CAP) and ARFI/SWE (Impulse Acoustic Radiation Force/Share Wave Elastography).

The diagnosis is important since it has proven that bariatric surgery is not only cost effective in cases of advanced fibrosis (f3), but also for obese patients with NASH, independently of the stage of fibrosis. Therefore, we must differentiate from the beginning the usefulness of these tests in the three diagnostic spectra of this disease: those that detect steatosis well, its evolution to NASH and fibrosis.

There are so many tests nowadays that are offered for the determination of steatosis and/or fibrosis of our patients, which will have to be adapted to each Center and to speak with the Hepatologist and the Radiologist when evaluating this disease in the best way possible. Thus, depending on the experience and availability of material they have, we may find variability among Hospitals regarding the imaging methods and biomarkers used in the diagnosis of NAFLD/NASH.

Keywords: Conventional Ultrasound (CUS), Computerized Tomography (CT), Magnetic Resonance Imaging (MRI, PDFF), Magnetic Resonance Spectroscopy (MRS), Magnetic Resonance Elastography (MRE), Transient Elastography (VCTE, CAP) and Impulse Acoustic Radiation Force/Share Wave Elastography (ARFI/SWE)

INTRODUCTION

The NAFLD and its evolution to NASH and later Fibrosis, which is complicated with Cirrhosis, Hepatic Failure and Hepatocarcinoma, that requires a transplant or end in the death of the patient, will shortly become one of the most prevalent diseases and that more resources health will need. Of course, it is the most common form of liver disease today [1, 2] affecting 80-100 million people in the United States [3]. We have arrived at this because of the pandemic that is Obesity, and the diseases that are related to it and that make up the Metabolic Syndrome, which as a pernicious vicious circle do nothing but feed back and take the patient to a point of no metabolic return.

The European Clinical Practice Guideline (EASL, EASD, EASO) for the management of NAFLD precisely defines this disease from the point of view of biopsy and image, which is the objective of this chapter. Thus, NAFLD is a mild condition that is characterized by excessive accumulation of liver fat (presence of steatosis in more than 5% of hepatocytes).

This percentage is calculated according to the histological analysis or a fat fraction of proton density (providing an approximate estimate of the volume fraction of fatty material in the liver) greater than 5.6%, evaluated well by magnetic resonance spectroscopy of protons (1H-MRS) or by selective magnetic resonance of fat/quantitative water (MRI) [4].

As the clinic is silent, if we do not think about it we will not be able to make the diagnosis, which is not indicated in the general population, but in obese or diabetic patients and who are at risk of liver disease. To make the diagnosis, we will begin with the imaging tests, where MR is the most accurate to determine the volume of liver fat, but it is expensive and not available to all centers.

Ultrasound is cheaper and accessible, but it has its limitations. Regarding the biological markers, we still do not have one that is totally reliable in the diagnosis of NASH, so we have to continue investigating, as well as in the different tests available [5]. Finally, we must continue to perform liver biopsy, an authentic gold-standard for the diagnosis of NASH, in patients at risk, either because they already have advanced disease or because of the more than predictable evolution to it.

The key to diagnosis is, therefore, in the non-invasive evaluation. Non-invasive markers should aim to: in the field of primary care, identify the risk of NAFLD in individuals with a high metabolic risk; in the field of secondary and tertiary care, identify individuals with a worse prognosis, for example, those with a severe NASH; monitor the progression of the disease; and predict the response to therapeutic interventions. If these objectives are achieved, the need for liver biopsies could be reduced [4].

Therefore, when a physician sees a patient with non-alcoholic fatty liver disease (NAFLD) in a clinical setting, three general clinical questions arise, which attempt to respond with imaging techniques: does my patient have NAFLD?; Does my patient have a nonalcoholic steatohepatitis (NASH)?; and Does my patient have advanced fibrosis? [6]. We must also ask ourselves which technique is best for each event, if it is cost efficient and what are its limitations.

The need for screening for NAFLD in the general population is highly questioned due to several factors: the high direct and indirect costs of the tests to be performed, the low predictive value of non-invasive tests, the risks of liver biopsy and the lack of effective treatments [7]. However, the progressive form of NAFLD (NASH), particularly when associated with advanced fibrosis, should be identified in at-risk patients (age> 50 years, type 2 diabetes mellitus or MetS), due to its prognostic implications. Similarly, although a family grouping occurs, it is generally not advisable to detect the family, with the exception of cases with defined hereditary diseases, for example, lysosomal acid lipase deficiency [4].

In the last two decades, enormous progress has been made in the evaluation of NAFLD by non-invasive images, techniques that receive more and more attention [6, 8]. Among these stand out (in addition to others in research that use biological markers and image): Ultrasound, Computerized Tomography, Magnetic Resonance Imaging (PDFF), Magnetic Resonance Spectroscopy, Magnetic Resonance Elastography, Transient Elastography (VCTE, CAP) and ARFI/SWE (Impulse Acoustic Radiation Force/Share Wave Elastography).

The available or developing imaging tests assess different properties of the tissue, including diffusion, texture, amount of fat, the amount of bonds in the fat and the stiffness of the liver [6]. Therefore it is important to know the pathophysiology of this disease to understand the new imaging techniques that are being developed and that associate the use of different biomarkers. These phenomena, together with the increase of cytokines and other substances, the damage of mitochondria, the different capacity of diffusion of gases by fatty particles, etc. have made possible the development of very promising techniques for the diagnosis of NAFDL and differentiate it from its progression to NASH.

The diagnosis is important since it has proven that bariatric surgery is not only cost effective in cases of advanced fibrosis (f3), but also for obese patients with NASH, independently of the stage of fibrosis [9]. Therefore, we must differentiate from the beginning the usefulness of these tests in the three diagnostic spectra of this disease: those that detect steatosis well, its evolution to NASH and fibrosis.

There are so many tests nowadays that are offered for the determination of steatosis and/or fibrosis of our patients, which will have to be adapted to each Center and to speak with the Hepatologist and the Radiologist when evaluating this disease in the best way possible. Thus, depending on the experience and availability of material they have, we may find variability among Hospitals regarding the imaging methods and biomarkers used in the diagnosis of NAFLD/NASH.

ECOGRAPHY

Ultrasound has always been used routinely in the preparation and study of our bariatric patients. And it is common for the radiologist to inform us of the presence of Fatty Liver, either with that term or with Hepatic Steatosis. Until now it was something like the "brand of the house" of every overweight patient. And it is because it is more accessible and cheaper than MRI, which is the benchmark.

Ultrasound has shown a sensitivity of 60 to 94% and a specificity of 84 to 95% in the detection of hepatic steatosis, being a first-line acceptable tool for the detection of steatosis in clinical practice, but cannot distinguish NASH of simple steatosis [8]. In addition, it does not reliably detect steatosis when it is <20% or in individuals with a high body mass index (> 40 kg/m^2). Despite its dependence on the operator, ultrasound reliably diagnoses moderate or severe steatosis and provides additional hepatobiliary information.

In this procedure, radiologists review the conventional brightness in the B-mode ultrasound images of the liver and the surrounding structures and evaluate the ultrasonographic characteristics known for fat content, such as the echogenicity of the liver in relation to the adjacent right kidney and darkness of Liver structures. From these qualitative characteristics, the presence and degree of hepatic steatosis can be inferred. The degree of steatosis can be reported using subjective terms ("mild, moderate, severe") or more formally using the CUS (Conventional Ultrasound) ordinal score designed to coincide with the ordinal scores used by pathologists to classify hepatic steatosis in histology [6].

The main advantages of the CUS is that it is a device available in any center, very well tolerated and safe, that is not expensive and that can be done with ultrasound from any manufacturer. On the other hand, among the main limitations is that the interpretation of the echographic characteristics of each patient is qualitative. In addition, other factors interfere in the test result, independently of the presence of hepatic steatosis, such as the characteristics of the patient (BMI, other liver diseases) and the test itself (observer, instruments such as ultrasound, transducer, probe) [6, 10].

Recent studies have shown that quantitative ultrasound may be superior to conventional ultrasound in detecting hepatic steatosis [11]. Ultrasound has also been used in different scores and studies to identify fatty liver and NASH, given its hyperechogenic and bright pattern [12]. Due to the limitations of other non-invasive tests, conventional ultrasound continues to be the diagnostic modality most commonly used to diagnose and qualify hepatic steatosis [6].

COMPUTERIZED TOMOGRAPHY (CT)

The CT scan is rarely used to look for NAFLD. In general, it is an incidental finding in an abdominal CT performed for another indication. The density of the liver/spleen ratio is typically used to detect hepatic steatosis on computed tomography. However, these studies are not of first indication for the evaluation of hepatic steatosis, since they expose patients to ionizing radiation [6].

In general, it is similar to Ultrasounds, and as limitations it has hemochromatosis and it does not distinguish Steatosis from NASH, and, as we have said, it also produces radiations [10]. It has been used in some studies, such as one on the improvement that bariatric surgery entailed on fatty liver, in which CT scans were performed before and one year after surgery [13].

MAGNETIC RESONANCE IMAGE (MRI)

MR is considered the "gold standard" of imaging techniques [14] and the most accurate method for determining NAFLD. It is also superior to ultrasound to detect steatosis of lesser amounts. It qualitatively and quantitatively identifies the fatty infiltration of the liver thanks to the fact that water and fat protons produce different frequencies in a magnetic field. The most widely used quantitative method is the so-called phase and out-of-phase image processing, in which the signal of the fat protons is added or subtracted, respectively, from the signal of the protons in the water. This makes it an accurate predictor of liver fat content compared to histological evaluation [15].

The term PDFF (Fraction of Fat of Proton Density) indicates a fundamental property of the liver tissue and represents the function of triglyceride protons visible by MR in the sum of triglycerides and water protons, and manages to estimate the hepatic fat content without using the spectroscopy. And it has the benefit that it can obtain a complete image of the liver, locating the area where we are going to measure the infiltration, since the liver fat is heterogeneous and is not evenly distributed, varying from one segment to another [6].

While it is very good at providing quantitative information on the accumulation of fat in the liver and although many MRI techniques have been developed to improve its performance in the diagnostic spectrum of NAFLD, these methods are limited in their ability to detect the coexistence of inflammation or fibrosis. In addition, MRI is expensive, time consuming and movement artifacts, such as breathing, can affect the quality of the image [10].

MRI can detect the quantitative decrease of fatty infiltration in the liver after bariatric surgery and, therefore, could be a valuable tool to monitor NAFLD/NASH after the operation [16]. MRI-PDFF is also useful for evaluating the response to treatment in early-phase NASH trials [17]. It also avoids confounding factors and is unaffected by the field strength of the scanner, patient factors (age, sex, body mass index and etiology of liver disease) and concomitant liver abnormalities such as iron overload or necroinflammation [18].

As a novelty in the use of MR in the search for NASH, DeMILI Test has emerged, as an online diagnostic service that allows, from a standard abdominal MRI, to obtain a report on the presence of NASH and liver fibrosis in a patient. It is accessed through a web platform and is based on two image biomarkers, FIBROmri and NASHmri. And, although it is a method still under evaluation, it already offers encouraging results with average areas under the curve (AUROC) of 0.83 for NASH and 0.85 for significant fibrosis [19].

Magnetic Resonance Spectroscopy (MRS)

It is today the technique of choice for the quantification of liver fat. In fact, and as we mentioned in the introduction, it is the one used in the European Guidelines for the definition of hepatic steatosis: fat fraction of proton density (providing an approximate estimate of the volume fraction of fatty material in the liver) greater than 5.6% [4]. With the right equipment and when the fat concentration is equal to or greater than 7.48%, it can be 100% accurate [20].

It consists of a very useful non-invasive technique that adds supplementary metabolic information to the anatomical anomalies that appear in radiological images of different diseases. It allows the evaluation, in vivo, of the molecular composition of the liver, and, although it fails in the detection of NASH, it has a high accuracy in the diagnosis of steatosis [8].

The precision of this quantitative method is achieved by separating the spectrum of the water curve from those of lipids and other metabolites, these curves expressed according to their resonance frequency measured in parts per million (ppm). But it has its limitations, since it requires specialized software, being also slow, complex and expensive. It remains, for all this, confined, at the moment, to research studies [10].

Elastography of Magnetic Resonance (MRE)

The search for a technique capable of differentiating steatosis from steatohepatitis seems to have found a possibility in Magnetic Resonance Elastography, in addition to other advantages. The fact that necroinflammation and fibrosis have similar effects could be the basis for differentiating NASH from NAFLD, but differentiates NASH from Fibrosis?. The limitation would be the excessive accumulation of iron [10]. It also seems that it would be profitable in the classification by stages of fibrosis, but, like other methods based on Magnetic Resonance, its availability is scarce in many centers, in addition to requiring an additional external validation [8].

The MRE, which was invented at the Mayo Clinic, is a non-invasive and effective method, which will require three stages to obtain results. In the first place, low frequency longitudinal waves, which deform the parenchyma, will be transmitted to the liver. These waves are transformed into transverse waves, called "cut or shear," which generate the data that is duly recorded. And finally, the analysis of these data, whose measurement, like the Transient Elastography by US, is quantified in kilopascals and that the equipment presents in the form of images.

This technique has a good correlation with liver biopsy, which has been the reason for different meta-analyzes [21, 22]. Thus, the efficacy of MRE in diagnosing fibrosis gave figures ranging between 0.87 and 0.99 under the AUROC curve, depending on whether it was stage of Fibrosis 1, 2, 3 or Cirrhosis, in both studies. And they concluded that the liver hardness measured by EMR increases with the degree of fibrosis. The higher the hardness, the more fibrosis [23].

On the other hand, it is superior on Transmission Elastography measured by Ultrasound, when it comes to achieving success, 94% in MRE over 84% in the US [24]. In addition, the volume of liver tissue that evaluates is much higher, being able to reach 250 cm3, compared to, at most, 20 cm3 of TE, reducing errors as heterogeneous as fibrosis may be, which makes the study be much more representative. Unlike ultrasound, Resonance Elastography is not affected by the presence of ascites or by the narrowness of the intercostal spaces [23].

But it remains the most important challenge to require this technique if it can differentiate steatosis from NASH [25]. Apparently it could do in the early stages of steatohepatitis, since the inflammation could have hardness similar to fibrosis. Thus, even in the absence of fibrosis, which in many cases can accompany necroinflammation from the beginning, MRE could have its usefulness in the early diagnosis of NASH.

Finally, an additional advantage of this method is the ability to perform a "multiparametric" scanning protocol by associating in the same session not only the study of fibrosis, but also the accumulation of fat or iron, adding other MR sequences. And although other authors find that this technique does not have the limitation of body mass, others believe that excessive obesity, together with the inability to sustain apnea, claustrophobia and biliary obstruction, can make testing difficult.

Transient Elastography Controlled by Vibration (VCTE)

Transient Elastography (FibroScan, Echosens, Paris, France) is a good tool for the calculation and non-invasive staging of Liver Stiffness Measurement (LSM). It will use the principles of ultrasound, applying low frequency cutting waves created by a vibratory probe at the level of an intercostal space that covers the liver. The elasticity, expressed in kilopascals, is determined by the elastic modulus calculated from the cutting wave velocity of the ultrasound signals.

The stiffness of the liver is determined with the value resulting from having made the calculations of the median of the 10 determinations made when applying the probe on the skin between the ribs of the patient, in the right part of the liver. Your measurements will place the patient at a certain level or degree of Fibrosis, which will have diagnostic implications, follow-up and, of course, treatment, being the average value for healthy people of 5.5 kPa.

When it is a value lower than 7 kPa it means that the level of progression is low, and it is recommended not to start with the treatment. Values between 7 and 9.4 kPa are evidence of moderate fibrosis or also called "level 2," and the patient should be tested with fibroscan regularly. Values between 9.4 and 12 kPa mean that the fibrosis is progressing and is "level 3," and with this result it is necessary to start treatment. When it exceeds 12 kPa, it means that the patient suffers from severe or "level 4" fibrosis, on the threshold of cirrhosis. This result indicates that the treatment or therapy is of an emergency nature.

Regardless of the cause that causes fibrosis, the mean areas under the curve (AUROC) were 0.84, 0.89 and 0.93 for the diagnosis of significant fibrosis, severe fibrosis and cirrhosis, respectively [26]. When the technique is analyzed in a wide series of cases and its comparison with the liver biopsy, it appears especially successful in the detection of more advanced fibrosis, such as F3 and F4, and with a moderate precision for the initial stages of fibrosis (F2). It is therefore a good method to differentiate advanced stages of hepatic fibrosis, compared to early stages [27].

It seems that obesity would be an adverse factor for the effectiveness of this technique, already with BMI above 28%. Therefore, to the conventional probe that reaches a depth of 25-65 mm (M-probe), a deeper probe (XL-probe) has been added that reaches up to 35-75 mm. Another adverse factor is the area analyzed, less than in other imaging techniques such as CT and any modality of MR, which analyze the entire liver. Likewise, situations such as necroinflammation of hepatocytes, cholestasis, elevated central venous pressure and postprandial conditions, can detract from this technique [10].

The greatest application that this method can contribute to the study of NAFLD would be to avoid performing liver biopsies, which according to the works could range from 45% of patients [26], to 60 or even 90% if fibrosis It is more advanced. At a fixed sensitivity, a cut LSM of 6.5 kPa excluded advanced fibrosis with a negative predictive value of 0.91, and a cut LSM of 12.1 kPa excluded cirrhosis with a negative predictive value of 0.99 [27].

Finally, the Controlled Attenuation Parameter (CAP) is nowadays used as a tool that can be useful in the assessment of liver fat. It is available in the latest devices for measuring the rigidity of the liver controlled by vibration (VCTE). The most current studies show that it can be used to detect hepatic steatosis, although it does not provide a reliable quantitative estimate of the liver fat content [6].

ARFI/SWE

ARFI is the Impulse of Acoustic Radiation Force. It is a form of elastography that calculates the elasticity of the liver from acoustic pulses of short duration of a fixed frequency directed to a region and is expressed in KPa. It is good for patients with very high BMI, even above 40 klgr/m2 [10]. Other authors suggest that the use of VCTE in combination with ARFI is highly specific to predict significant fibrosis and may decrease the need for a liver biopsy.

The SWE (supersonic images of cutting waves) is a new technique of ultrasound elastography that has been used for the assessment of liver fibrosis. It has the advantage that being an evaluation in the form of a fan will value a larger region of the liver. It has also been used in the assessment of different chronic liver diseases, being superimposable to other elastographic techniques, such as VCTE and ARFI, and how they are fast, reliable and simple. But it has not appreciably evaluated steatosis in patients with NAFLD [10].

We can conclude by stating that ARFI is a promising image modality to detect advanced fibrosis in patients with liver disease related to obesity. And there are authors who believe that SWE and ARFI provide a better and more reliable estimate of liver fibrosis than VCTE [6].

MONITORING AND CONTROL

When deciding which is the best follow-up for our patients, we must take into account many aspects. Both the risk that the liver disease may progress to cirrhosis, and the workload of all specialists related to the disease, as well as the cost of imaging procedures, are issues to consider. Perhaps for all this, to date, there is no consensus on what would be the best follow-up protocol for these patients. What is agreed is that the surveillance of these patients should include routine biochemical parameters, noninvasive evaluation of fibrosis (imaging techniques, among others) and study of associated comorbidities.

Thus, patients with NAFLD who do not have worsening of their metabolic risk factors, that is, who are stable, should be monitored every 2 or 3 years. However, the control should be annual in those patients who have NASH or Fibrosis. And every 6 months if the evolution of the disease has reached cirrhosis. In these cases, and on an individual basis, the repeat of the biopsy at 5 years may be indicated.

COMPARISON OF THE DIFFERENT TECHNIQUES

Table 1. Efficacy of the imaging tests in the detection of Steatosis, NASH and Fibrosis

Effectiveness of the evidenceof image in NAFLD	Steatosis	Nash	Fibrosis
ECOGRAPHY	+	-	-
CT	+	-	-
RMI	+	-	+
RMS	+	-	+
RME	+	-	+
VCTE	+	-	+
ARFI	-	-	+

Table 2. Limitations of these techniques

	Radiation	Obesity	Claustrophobia	Cost	Time	Artefactors	Operator Dependent	Hemosiderosis
US	-	++	-	+	-	-	+++	-
CT	+++	-	-	++	-	-	-	-
RMI	-	-	+++	++	++	++	-	++
RMS	-	-	+++	+++	+++	++	-	++
RME	-	-	+++	+++	+++	++	-	++
UCTE	-	+	-	+	+	-	-	-
ARFI	-	-/+	-	+	+	-	-	-

Table 3. Comparison of elastographic techniques

Elastography	Cost	Accuracy	Problems
VCTE	+	++	Obesity Cirrhosis
ARFI/SWE	+	++	Obesity Cirrhosis
RME	+++	+++	Hemosiderosis

REFERENCES

[1] Ooi, GJ, Burton, PR, Bayliss, J, Raajendiran, A, Earnest, A, Laurie, C, Kemp, WW, McLean, CA, Roberts, SK, Watt, MJ, Brown, WA. 2019. "Effect of Body Mass Index, Metabolic Health and Adipose Tissue Inflammation on the Severity of Non-Alcoholic Fatty Liver Disease in Bariatric Surgical Patients: a Prospective Study." *Obesity Surgery* 29 (1): 99-108. doi: 10.1007/s11695-018-3479-2.

[2] Tan, CH, Al-Kalifah, N, Ser, KH, Lee, YC, Chen, JC, Lee, WJ. 2018. "Long-term effect of bariatric surgery on resolution of nonalcoholic steatohepatitis (NASH): An external validation and application of a

clinical NASH score." *Surgery of Obesity and Related Disease.* 14 (10): 1600-06. Accessed June 6, 2018. doi: 10.1016/j.soard.2018.05.024.

[3] Alkhouri, N. and Feldstein, A. E. 2016. "Noninvasive diagnosis of nonalcoholic fatty liver disease: are we there yet?." *Metabolism* 65 (8): 1087-95. Accessed February 2, 2016. doi: 10.1016/j.metabol.2016.01.013.

[4] Marchesini, G. et al. 2016. "EASL-EASD-EASO Clinical Practice Guidelines for the management of non-alcoholic fatty liver disease." *Journal of Hepatology* 64: 1388-402.

[5] López, IC, Aroca, FG, Bernal, MDF, Mompean, JAL, Bernal, ÁB, Martínez, AMH, Barba, EM, Velasco, JAN, Paricio, PP. 2017. "Utility of the ELF Test for Detecting Steatohepatitis in Morbid Obese Patients with Suspicion of Nonalcoholic Fatty Liver Disease." *Obesity Surgery* 27 (9): 2347-53. doi: 10.1007/s11695-017-2606-9.

[6] Loomba, R. 2018. "Role of imaging-based biomarkers in NAFLD: Recent advances in clinical application and future research directions." *Journal of Hepatology* 68: 1296-304.

[7] Chalasani, N, Younossi, Z, Lavine, JE, Charlton, M, Cusi, K, Rinella, M, Harrison, SA, Brunt, EM, Sanyal, AJ. 2018. "The Diagnosis and Management of Nonalcoholic Fatty Liver Disease: Practice Guidance from the American Association for the Study of Liver Diseases." *Journal of Hepatology* 67 (1): 328-357.

[8] Gallego-Durán, R. et al. 2016. "Imaging biomarkers for steatohepatitis and fibrosis detection in non-alcoholic fatty liver disease." *Scientific Reports 6*, Article Number: 31421.

[9] Klebanoff, MJ, Corey, KE, Chhatwal, J, Kaplan, LM, Chung, RT, Hur, C. 2017. "*Bariatric surgery for nonalcoholic steatohepatitis: A clinical and cost-effectiveness analysis.*" 65 (4): 1156-64. Accessed February 21, 2017. doi: 10.1002/hep.28958.

[10] Valle Tovo, C, Zambam de Mattos, A, Coral, G, Schild Branco, F, Suwa, E and Alves de Mattos, A. 2015. "Noninvasive imaging assessment of non-alcoholic fatty liver disease: Focus on liver

scintigraphy." *World Journal of Gastroenterology* 21 (15): 4432-39. Accessed April 21, 2015. doi: 10.3748/wjg.v21.i15.4432.

[11] Lin, SC, Heba, E, Wolfson, T et al. 2015. "Noninvasive diagnosis of nonalcoholic fatty liver disease and quantification of liver fat using a new quantitative ultrasound technique." *Clinical Gastroenterology and Hepatoly* 13: 1337-45.

[12] Goossens, N et al. 2016. "Nonalcoholic Steatohepatitis Is Associated with Increased Mortality in Obese Patients Undergoing Bariatric Surgery." *Clinical Gastroenterology and Hepatology*. 14 (11): 1619-28. Accessed October 20, 2015. doi: 10.1016/j.cgh. 2015.10.010.

[13] Uehara, D, Seki, Y, Kakizaki, S, Horiguchi, N, Tojima, H, Yamazaki, Y, Sato, K, Yamada, M, Uraoka, T, Kasama, K. 2019. "Long-term Results of Bariatric Surgery for Non-Alcoholic Fatty Liver Disease/Non-alcoholic Steatohepatitis Treatment in Morbidly Obese Japanese Patients." *Obesity Surgery* 29 (4): 1195-201. doi: 10.1007/s11695-018-03641-2.

[14] Cantero, I et al. 2019. "Ultrasound/Elastography techniques, lipidomic and blood markers compared to Magnetic Resonance Imaging in non-alcoholic fatty liver disease adults." *International Journal of Medical Sciences*. 16 (1): 75-83. doi: 10.7150/ijms.28044.

[15] Tang A, Tan J, Sun M, Hamilton G, Bydder M, Wolfson T, Gamst AC, Middleton M, Brunt EM, Loomba R, et al. 2013. "Nonalcoholic fatty liver disease: MR imaging of liver proton density fat fraction to assess hepatic steatosis." *Radiology* 267: 422-31.

[16] Hedderich, DM, Hasenberg, T, Haneder, S, Schoenberg, SO, Kücükoglu, Ö, Canbay, A, Otto, M. 2017. "Effects of Bariatric Surgery on Non-alcoholic Fatty Liver Disease: Magnetic Resonance Imaging Is an Effective, Non-invasive Method to Evaluate Changes in the Liver Fat Fraction." *Obesity Surgery* 27 (7): 1755-62. doi: 10.1007/s11695-016-2531-3.

[17] Caussy, C, Reeder, SB, Sirlin, CB and Loomba, R. 2018. "Noninvasive, Quantitative Assessment of Liver Fat by MRI-PDFF as an Endpoint in NASH Trials." *Hepatology*. 68 (2): 763-72. doi: 10.1002/hep.29797.

[18] Younossi, ZM, Loomba, R et al. 2018. "Diagnostic Modalities for Nonalcoholic Fatty Liver Disease, Nonalcoholic Steatohepatitis, and Associated Fibrosis." *Hepatology* 68 (1): 349-60. doi: 10.1002/hep.29721.

[19] Wong, VW et al. 2018. "Noninvasive biomarkers in NAFLD and NASH - current progress and future promise." *Nat Rev Gastroenterol Hepatol.* 15 (8): 461-78. doi: 10.1038/s41575-018-0014-9.

[20] Roldan Valdez, E, Favila, R, Martinez López, M et al. 2008. "Imaging techniques for assessing hepatic fat content in nonalcoholic fatty liver disease." *Ann Hepatol*, 7: 212-20.

[21] Wang, QB, Zhu, H, Liu, LL et al. 2012. "Performance of magnetic resonance elastography and diffusion-weighted imaging for the staging of hepatic fibrosis: A meta-analysis." *Hepatology,* 56: 237-39.

[22] Su, LN, Guo, SL, Li, BX et al. 2014. "Diagnostic value of magnetic resonance elastography for detecting and staging of hepatic fibrosis: A meta-analysis." *Clin Radiol*, 69: 545-52.

[23] Stoopen-Rometti, M et al. 2017. "Diagnosis and quantification of fibrosis, steatosis and hepatosiderosis by means of multiparametric magnetic resonance." *Journal of Gastroenterology of Mexico*. 82 (1): 32-45. doi.org/10.1016/j.rgmx.2016.06.001.

[24] Huwart, L, Sempoux, C, Vicaut, E et al. 2008. "Magnetic resonance elastography for the noninvasive staging of liver fibrosis." *Gastroenterology,* 135: 32-40.

[25] Ajmera, V, Loomba, R. 2018. "Can Elastography Differentiate Isolated Fatty Liver from Nonalcoholic Steatohepatitis?." *Semin Liver Dis.* 38 (1): 14-20. Accessed February 22, 2018. doi: 10.1055/s-0037-1618587.

[26] Tapper, EB et al. 2016. "The Performance of Vibration Controlled Transient Elastography in a US Cohort of Patients With Nonalcoholic Fatty Liver Disease." *American Journal of Gastroenterology.* 111 (5): 677-84. Accessed March 15, 2016. doi: 10.1038/ajg.2016.49.

[27] Siddiqui, MS et al. 2019. "Vibration-Controlled Transient Elastography to Assess Fibrosis and Steatosis in Patients with Nonalcoholic Fatty Liver Disease." *Clinical Gastroenterology and*

Hepatology. 17 (1): 156-63. Accessed April 26, 2018. doi: 10.1016/j.cgh.2018.04.043.

In: Liver Steatosis and Bariatric Surgery ISBN: 978-1-53616-444-2
Editors: Jaime Ruiz-Tovar et al.

Chapter 7

MR SPECTROSCOPY AND QUANTIFICATION OF INTRAHEPATOCITARY LIPID CONTENT

***Jaime Ruiz-Tovar**, MD, PhD and Carolina Llavero*†**
Obesity Unit, Garcilaso Clinic, Madrid, Spain

ABSTRACT

Currently, the standard procedure used to evaluate hepatic steatosis is the liver biopsy. This is an invasive practice that presents inherent risks. Increasing evidence suggests that Magnetic resonance imaging (MRI) and MR spectroscopy (MRS) may represent an accurate method to determine the hepatic lipid content.

In this chapter we will review the actual evidence about the use of MR spectroscopy to evaluate liver steatosis and non-alcoholic fatty liver disease (NAFLD).

Keywords: liver steatosis, magnetic resonance, spectroscopy, percentage of lipid content

* Corresponding Author's Email: jruiztovar@gmail.com.
† Carolina Llavero, RN.

INTRODUCTION

Nonalcoholic fatty liver disease (NAFLD) is characterized by lipid deposit in the hepatocytes of the liver parenchyma, exceeding the 5% of the liver weight. NAFLD includes a spectrum of disorders ranging from simple steatosis, a relatively benign condition, to nonalcoholic steatohepatitis (NASH) and pericellular or perisinusoidal fibrosis. In some cases, these entities might lead to a cirrhosis stage, similar to the observed in alcoholic hepatitis. The mechanism of NAFLD is still unknown, but involves the development of insulin resistance, inflammatory cytokines and oxidative stress [1, 2].

NAFLD is strongly associated with obesity, mainly with central one, and has become the most common liver disorder in Western countries [3]. The prevalence of NAFLD, in any degree, is estimated around 70% in obese subjects and up to 95% in morbidly obese patients [4]. Among patients undergoing bariatric surgery, liver steatosis is the most common degree of the disease, appearing NASH in about 25% of the cases and cirrhosis in 1-3% [5].

The diagnosis of NAFLD is usually made after an incidental discovery of unexplained elevation of liver enzyme levels or when steatosis is observed on imaging. Currently, the standard procedure used to evaluate hepatic steatosis is the histopathological examination of cross-liver sections and the semi-quantitative estimation of the percentage of hepatocytes containing macrovesicular fat. This is an invasive practice that presents inherent risks [1]. Despite there are several series in literature with an elevated number of patients undergoing a liver biopsy during bariatric surgery, without showing any morbidity related with the biopsy [6], for posterior monitoring of the liver status it is necessary to perform a percutaneous liver biopsy, implying an invasive procedure. Moreover, histological examination of cross-liver sections and the determination of the percentage of hepatocytes containing macrovesicular fat, only provides a two-dimensional estimation of a particular biopsy and is subject to inter-individual visual evaluation depending on the pathologist's training, which usually results in overestimation of the liver fat content [7, 8]. Therefore, it is essential to establish new non-invasive approaches to accurately determine the hepatic fat concentration, allowing the correct diagnosis and monitoring of steatosis.

The liver cell injury and intra-hepatocellular accumulation of lipids can be also evaluated by noninvasive tests. Increasing evidence suggests that Magnetic resonance imaging (MRI) and MR spectroscopy (MRS) may represent an accurate method to determine the hepatic lipid content, comparable to the liver biopsy to measure and follow up the fatty liver disease. Thus, they have been postulated as potential screening tools for patients at risk of liver steatosis, such as morbidly obese patients [8].

MRI represents a potential non-invasive technique for assessing hepatic steatosis in three-dimensions. MRS is a suitable method to quantify hepatic lipid content, as the values obtained by MRS are directly related to the molecular triglyceride content [9, 10]. One of the main advantages of using spectroscopy instead of biopsy is that it can be performed contemporaneously with MR imaging and the sampling volumes are larger than the obtained in liver biopsy avoiding misinterpretations if the fat liver distribution is heterogeneous [11, 12].

Liver Steatosis and Bariatric Surgery

Bariatric surgery achieves an improvement or even complete resolution of NAFLD in morbidly obese patients. This fact has been demonstrated after Roux-en–Y gastric bypass (RYGBP), adjustable gastric banding and malabsorptive procedures (duodenal switch and biliopancreatic diversion) and sleeve gastrectomy (SG) [5, 13-16].

Liver steatosis regression has been associated with an improvement in the lipid profile, which is more likely to occur after malabsorptive techniques. However, a study of our group demonstrated a significant reduction of triglyceride levels and an increase of HDL-cholesterol 12 months after undergoing a sleeve gastrectomy, achieving both parameters values within the normal range. Therefore, an improvement of liver steatosis was observed, as expected. Our results were similar to those reported after Roux-en-Y gastric bypass (90-95% of resolution of the steatosis) [17, 18].

MR Imaging and MR Spectroscopy

The MRI protocol performed at our institution included preoperative evaluation 2 weeks prior to surgery and postoperative evaluation at 6 months Postoperatively.

Axial T1-wi dual gradient-echo (TR/TE, 122 ms/5-2 ms; flip angle, 80°; slice thickness, 6 mm; matrix 256 × 256). In addition axial breath hold three dimensional (3D) T1-weighted high resolution isotropic volume examination (THRIVE) (TR/TE, 4/2 ms; flip angle, 10°; reconstructed slice thickness, 2 mm; matrix, 256 × 256) was acquired for volumetric analysis.

Before spectroscopy, for a better voxel placement, fast T2 single shot TSE sequences (TR/TE, 611/100 ms; flip angle 90°, slice thickness/GAP, 9/0.9 mm) were acquired in coronal, sagital and axial planes. MRS was acquired with the single-voxel technique, two voxels were located in different regions within the left and right hepatic lobes to provide a more generalized distribution of fat within the liver. The average voxel volume was of 30 x 30 x 30 mm and 20 x 20 x 20 mm for the voxels located in the right lobe and left hepatic lobe, respectively. The voxel was located avoiding blood vessels, the gall bladder, and fatty tissue. After volume-selective autoshimming, the spectra were obtained with a point-resolved spectroscopy (PRESS) technique (TR/TE/scans = 2000 ms/35 ms/64) without water suppression. Each spectrum consisted of 1,024 complex data points in the time domain with a spectral width of 2,000 Hz. Chemical shift was placed relative to the water signal intensity.

Spectra were analyzed offline in the time domain using the AMARES algorithm included in the MRUI software package as described previously. The relative lipid content was defined by following the formulae [19]:

$$RLC = S_{lipid}/(S_{lipid} + S_{water})$$

For volumetric analysis, manual volumetric segmentations of the liver were performed by manual tracing of the liver on volumetric sequences in the axial plane avoiding the gall bladder and main hepatic vessels at a dedicated workstation (Advantage Workstation, Version 4.3; GE Healthcare Europe, Buc, France).

Steatosis by MRS was determined as absent when detected percentage of lipid content (PLC) was lower than 5%, mild when lower than 10%, moderate when 10-30% and severe when >30%, as described in literature [20-23].

EVALUATION OF LIVER STEATOSIS AFTER SG, ASSESSED BY MR SPECTROCOPY

Indication for undergoing SG was presenting a body mass index (BMI) $\geq$40 Kg/m^2 or BMI $\geq$35 Kg/m^2 with comorbidities. Patients presenting a daily alcohol intake of more than 20 g per day, chronic hepatitis B or C virus infection, hepatotoxic drugs intake or other known liver diseases, presence of pacemaker or any metallic implant not compatible with MR, and claustrophobia, are not evaluated with MR spectroscopy.

We performed a prospective observational study evaluating liver steatosis, as measured by MR spectroscopy in 23 patients undergoing SG, with a mean age of 47.6 ± 10.6 years and a mean BMI 47.6 ± 6.7 Kg/m^2. Six months after surgery, MR spectroscopy was repeated. At that time, mean BMI 32.2 ± 5.1 Kg/m^2, with a mean excess weight loss of 68.2 ± 18.6%.

Mean preoperative hepatic volume was 1999.9 ± 436.2 ml and 6 months after surgery the liver volume significantly decreased to 1568 ± 170.3 ml ($p = 0.005$). Mean preoperative percentage of lipid content (PLC) was 14.2 ± 15.4% and 6 months after surgery these values decreased to 4.3 ± 3.2% ($p = 0.007$). A significant reduction of steatosis grade was observed, with disappearance of preoperative steatosis in 54.9% of the patients. Six months after surgery, 91.3% of the patients did not present any grade of steatosis.

In our study, we observed a preoperative steatosis incidence calculated with MRS of 63.6%. This steatosis rate is similar to the one observed by some authors, though other reports have shown higher prevalence that could vary from 65 to 80%. The steatosis grade was probably lower among our patients, as all of them followed a strict preoperative diet and a weight loss of at least a 5% of their overweight was a necessary condition to undergo the sleeve gastrectomy as bariatric procedure. It has been demonstrated that establishing strict dietary treatments with a total caloric intake of less than 1000 kcal / day between 2 and 8 weeks before surgery, in order to maximize weight loss during this period of time, result in a reduction of the surgical risk. This weight loss is associated with a reduction of hepatomegalia secondary to liver steatosis. We have observed a positive correlation between hepatic lipid content assessed by MRS and hepatic volume, suggesting that the hepatic volume loss observed after surgery is related to the decrease in the hepatic lipid content, as it has been previously reported in patients undergoing bariatric surgery.

Alterations of AST and ALT are the most frequent conditions found in NAFLD in morbidly obese patients [2], similar to our results. Notwithstanding, Dixon et al. [24] reported that changes in aminotransferase concentrations seems not to predict changes in steatosis. In the same line, a recent study observed a significant reduction of steatosis after bariatric surgery, documented with liver biopsy, but without correlation with AST or ALT levels. In our series, we observed a correlation between liver enzymes and PLC in the preoperative determinations, but the decrease of liver enzymes or the postoperative values did not show any correlation with PLC decrease or postoperative PLC values. Liver steatosis rate in morbidly obese patients ranges between 65-80%, but steatohepatitis appears in only 25% of the case. Hepatocyte fat infiltration might lead to a certain degree of inflammation and cytolysis, but this is especially relevant in severe steatosis grades. Thus, in the preoperative determinations of our series, with more than 25% of patients presenting severe steatosis, more steatohepatitis would be present and therefore a correlation with liver enzymes is possible. Postoperatively, steatosis remains in few patients and just in mild grade with probably absence of steatohepatitis, preventing a positive correlation between both entities [1].

Evaluation of Liver Steatosis after RYGB, Assessed by MR Spectrocopy

A similar study to the previously reported one on patients undergoing SG, was conducted on patients undergoing Roux-en-Y gastric bypass. Inclusion and exclusion criteria were similar. 21 patients were included, with a mean age of 48 ± 10.6 years and a mean BMI of 47.1 ± 10.5 Kg/m^2. Six months after surgery, mean BMI was 31.7 ± 4.9 Kg/m^2 with a mean excess weight loss of 69.3 ± 17.7%. Preoperative percentage of lipid content (P^LC) was 13.3 ± 10.4%, with a significant decrease up to 3.5 ± 2.6% after surgery. Preoperatively, 70% of the patients presented liver statosis at any degree, while after surgery a complete remission of steatosis was observed in all the cases, excepting one patient with steatosis grade III, decreasing to a grade I [25, 26].

Comparing these results with those obtained after SG, these are quite similar, concluding equivalent results at 6 months after surgery.

Limitations of MR Spectroscopy

The knowledge of percentage of lipid content is relevant, so long it is part of NAFLD and is associated with the progression to NASH or even cirrhosis. However, the disappearnace of liver steatosis after bariatric surgery does not necessary imply the remission of NASH and even less the regression of cirrhosis. Thus, to evaluate these issues, MR spectroscopy is not probably the most accurate method. Serum biomarkers can be helpful, despite their value is still controversial. Liver biopsy remains the gold standard to assess NASH and its evolution after bariatric surgery.

CONCLUSION

After bariatric surgery, a significant reduction of liver steatosis is observed, as demonstrated by a statistically significant reduction in the percentage of intrahepatocitary lipids and liver volume, determined by MR spectros and MRI. These imaging techniques can be considered as noninvasive, accurate methods for monitoring liver steatosis in morbidly obese patients undergoing bariatric surgery.

REFERENCES

[1] Wilkins T, Tadkod A, Hepburn I, et al. Nonalcoholic fatty liver disease: diagnosis and management. *Am. Fam. Physician.* 2013;88:35-42.

[2] Alves de Carvalho MS, Coelho Cabral P, Kruze Grande de Arruda I, et al. Risk factors associated with hepatic steatosis; a study in patients in the Northeast Brazil. *Nutr. Hosp.* 2012;27:1344-1350.

[3] Clark JM, Brancati FL, Diehl AM. Nonalcoholic fatty liver disease. *Gastroenterology* 2002;122:1649-1657.

[4] Clark JM, Alkhuraishi AR, Solga SF, et al. Roux-en-Y gastric bypass improves liver histology in patients with non-alcoholic fatty liver disease. *Obes. Res.* 2005;13:1180-1186.

[5] Pillai AA, Rinella ME. Non-alcoholic fatty liver disease: is bariatric surgery the answer? *Clin. Liver Dis.* 2009;13:689-710.

[6] Subichin M, Clanton J, Makuszewski M, et al. Liver disease in the morbidly obese: a review of 1000 consecutive patients undergoing weight loss surgery. *Surg. Obes. Relat. Dis.* 2015;11:137-141.

[7] Jimenez-Aguero R, Emparanza JI, Beguiristain A, et al. Novel equation to determine the hepatic triglyceride concentration in humans by MRI: diagnosis and monitoring of NAFLD in obese patients before and after bariatric surgery. *BMC Medicine* 2014;12:137-151.

[8] Younossi ZM, Gramlich T, Liu YC, et al. Nonalcoholic fatty liver disease: assessment of variability in pathologic interpretations. *Mod. Pathol.* 1998;11:560-565.

[9] Reeder SB, Cruite I, Hamilton G, et al. Quantitative assessment of liver fat with magnetic resonance imaging and spectroscopy. *J. Magn. Reson. Imaging* 2011;34:729-749.

[10] Tang A, Tan J, Sun M, et al. Nonalcoholic fatty liver disease: MR imaging of liver proton density fat fraction to assess hepatic steatosis. *Radiology* 2013;267:422-431.

[11] Chan DC, Watts GF, Ng TWK, et al. Measurement of liver fat by magnetic resonance imaging: Relationships with body fat distribution, insulin sensitivity and plasma lipids in healthy men. *Diabetes Obes. Metab*. 2006;8:698-702.

[12] Ishii M, Yoshioka Y, Ishida W, et al. Liver fat content measured by magnetic resonance spectroscopy at 3.0 tesla independently correlates with plasminogen activator inhibitor-1 and body mass index in type 2 diabetic subjects. *Tohoku J. Exp. Med.* 2005;206:23-30.

[13] Weiner RA. Surgical treatment of non-alcoholic steatohepatitis and non-alcoholic fatty liver disease. *Dig. Dis*. 2010;28:274-279.

[14] Johansson HE, Haenni A, Zethelius B. Platelet counts and liver enzymes after bariatric surgery. *J. Obes*. 2013;Article ID 567984.

[15] Tai CM, Huang CK, Hwang JC, et al. Improvement of nonalcoholic fatty liver disease after bariatric surgery in morbidly obese Chinese patients. *Obes. Surg*. 2012;22:1016-1021.

[16] Sakçak M, Avsar MF, Hamamci EO, et al. Comparison of early and late changes in immunoglobulins and acute phase reactants after laparoscopic adjustable gastric banding in patients with morbid obesity. *Obes. Surg*. 2010;20:610-615.

[17] Weiner RA. Surgical treatment of non-alcoholic steatohepatitis and non-alcoholic fatty liver disease. *Dig. Dis*. 2010;28:274-279.

[18] Alsina ME, Ruiz-Tovar J, Bernabeu A. Evolution of Liver Steatosis Quantified by MR Imaging and MR Spectroscopy, in Morbidly Obese Patients Undergoing Sleeve Gastrectomy: Short-Term Outcomes. *Obes. Surg*. 2017; 27:1724-1728.

[19] van Werven JR, Marsman HA, Nederveen AJ, et al. Assessment of hepatic steatosis in patients undergoing liver resection: comparison of US, CT, T1-weighted dual-echo MR imaging, and point-resolved 1H MR spectroscopy. *Radiology* 2010;256:159-168.

[20] Moreno-Pérez O, Portilla J, Escoín C, et al. Impact of vitamin D insufficiency on insulin homeostasis and beta cell function in nondiabetic male HIV-infected patients. *HIV Med.* 2013;14:540-548.

[21] Ma X, Holalkere N-S, Kambadakone R A, et al. Imaging-based quantification of hepatic fat: methods and clinical applications. *Radiographics* 2009; 29:1253-1277.

[22] Machann J, Thamer C, Schnoedt B, et al. Hepatic lipid accumulation in healthy subjects: A comparative study using spectral fat-selective MRI and volume-localized 1H-MR spectroscopy. *Magn. Reson. Med.* 2006; 55:913-917.

[23] Thomas EL, Hamilton G, Patel N, et al. Hepatic triglyceride content and its relation to body adiposity: a magnetic resonance imaging and proton magnetic resonance spectroscopy study. *Gut* 2005;54:122-127.

[24] Dixon JB, Bhathal PS, O'Brien PE. Weight loss and non-alcoholic fatty liver disease: falls in gamma-glutamyl transferase concentrations are associated with histologic improvement. *Obes. Surg.* 2006;10:1278-1286.

[25] Vargas V, Allende H, Lecube A, et al. Surgically induced weight loss by gastric bypass improves non alcoholic fatty liver disease in morbid obese patients. *World J. Hepatol.* 2012;4:382-388.

[26] Pontiroli AE, Benetti A, Folini L, et al. Other aspects of bariatric surgery: liver steatosis, ferritin and cholesterol metabolism. *Nutr. Hosp.* 2013;28:104-108.

In: Liver Steatosis and Bariatric Surgery
Editors: Jaime Ruiz-Tovar et al.
ISBN: 978-1-53616-444-2

Chapter 8

BIOCHEMICAL MARKERS

Soledad García-Gómez-Heras**, *MD, PhD
Department of Histology, Rey Juan Carlos University,
Madrid, Spain

ABSTRACT

Liver biopsy, although "gold standard" for the diagnosis of NAFLD/NASH, has some limitations. Nowadays, biochemical markers are an alternative less invasive or noninvasive tests and have the important characteristics of diagnostic tests. They focus on the specific pathways involved in the progression of disease: hepatocyte death or apoptosis, inflammation, fibrosis and oxidative stress.

Keywords: NASH-disgnosis, NAFLD, biochemical markers, non invasive test

* Corresponding Author's Email: soledad.garcia@urjc.es.

INTRODUCTION

The current "*gold standard*" for the diagnosis and stratification of NAFLD is liver biopsy. It can determine necroinflammatory activity, degree of steatosis, and extent of fibrosis. But liver biopsy has some limitations as we have exposed in the other chapter: sample size, bleeding, pain, etc. so it is a resource that cannot be used routinely.

With the increasing incidence of NAFLD, we need to do regular control for NAFLD progression, evaluation of hepatic steatosis, NASH and advanced fibrosis.

The knowledge of whether a patient has simple steatosis or NASH is very important prognostically. Patients with NASH can progress to cirrhosis and therefore should be more actively managed to try and prevent disease progression.

This situation has led to the search of alternative less invasive or noninvasive tests to assess NAFLD. Nowadays, biochemical markers have the important characteristics of diagnostic tests: good cost-effectiveness, ease, and reproducibility. Their presence and level are not liver specific but they have been associated with pathophysiologic liver disease processes (Pepe et al. 2001, Ruiz-Tovar et al. 2019, Tsai et al., 2018).

Several biomarkers have been proposed for the evaluation of hepatic steatosis, the prediction and progression of NASH and significant/advanced fibrosis. Next we expose some.

LABORATORY DATA

They included platelet count, alanine aminotranspherase (ALT), aspartate aminotranspherase (AST), insulin and albumin levels, in order to analyze the following formulas:

- Hepatic Steatosis Index (HSI) = 8 x ALT/AST + BMI (+2 if T2D yes, +2 if female)

- Liver Fat Score (LFS) = -2.89 + 1.18 x Metabolic Syndrome (Yes: 1; No:0) + 0.45 x T2D (Yes: 2; No:0) + 0.15 Insulin in uU/l + 0.04 x AST in U/L – 0.94 x AST/ALT
- AST to Platelet Ratio Index (APRI) = (AST/ALT x100) / Platelets (10^9/L)
- Fibrosis-4 (FIB-4) = (Age (years) x AST) / (Platelets x ALT)
- Non-alcoholic fatty liver Disease-Fibrosis Score (NAFLDFS) = -1.675 + 0.037 x age + 0.094 x BMI + 1.13 x Diabetes (Yes: 1; No:0) + 0.99 x AST/ALT – 0.013 x Platelet – 0.66 x Albumin.

BIOMARKERS FOCUS ON THE SPECIFIC PATHWAYS INVOLVED IN THE PROGRESSION OF DISEASE

Biomarkers Focus on Hepatocyte Death or Apoptosis

- Serum Cytokeratin 18 (CK18) levels.

Describe initialy by Feldstein et al. in 2009, reporting circulating serum levels of CK-18 to be predictive of NASH in patients with NAFLD. It is by far the one that has been the most widely investigated (Castera et al., 2019).

CK18 fragments are major intermediate filaments of hepatocytes. CK-18 fragments come from apoptosis of hepatocytes accomplished by the enzyme caspase 3 and can be measured in serum by immunoassay.

Serum CK18 levels correlate with histologic changes and reflect severity of NASH. Studies have shown its high specificity for NAFLD and fibrosis (Cusi K, et al., 2104; Tsai et al., 2018).

- Fibroblast growth factor 21 (FGF21), showed greater association with disease progression (Shen J, et al. 2012).
- CK18-M65 (uncleaved CK18), with strong accuracy in predicting NASH (Younossi et al., 2008).

Markers of Inflammation

- Ferritin
- C-reactive protein (CRP)

They are nonspecific markers of inflammation that have been shown to be associated with NASH (Hui et al. 2004; Musso et al., 2011; Targher et al., 2006).

- Adipocytokines. They are associated with presence and severity of disease. Studies have shown that low levels of adiponectin and high levels of tumor necrosis factor-a (TNF-a) are associated with higher levels of liver damage (Jarrar et al., 2008; Hui et al., 2004 b)
- Interleukin-6 and interleukin-8. Some studies have shown that are strongly correlated with NASH (Abiru et al., 2006; Ajmera et al., 2017; Wieckowska et al., 2008).

Biomarkers of Fibrosis

- Serum aminotransferases, they are not useful in diagnosing fibrosis but levels often decrease when fibrosis worsens. An AST/ALT ratio greater than 1 has been shown to be predictive of fibrosis because of impaired AST clearance (Williams et al., 1988).
- Hyaluronic acid (HA) production increases in fibrosis and its clearance decreases in advanced liver disease. Studies have reported good correlation of high HA levels with advanced fibrosis. However, different cutoff values were used, rendering interpretation difficult (Hartley et al., 206; Kaneda et al., 2006; Piperno et al., 1998; Suzuki et al., 2005).

Markers of Oxidative Stress

Measurements of serum markers of oxidative stress are difficult because of their volatile nature but they are of interest becausse oxidative stress contributes to the pathogenesis of NASH; oxidized low-density lipoprotein, malonaldehyde, and thiobarbituric acid reactive substances have been evaluated in predicting NASH but results have been conflicting (Yesilova et al., 2005; Chalasani et al., 2004).

None of the available biomarkers have high sensitivity and specificity able to differentiate NASH from simple steatosis but they provide important information that require a critical interpretation of the results. For this reason, the use of imaging tests further complements the information available. It is desirable to look for the ideal combination between biomarkers and imaging tests (ultrasonography, computed tomography, elastographic techniques, magnetic resonance) (Ruiz-Tovar et al. 2019).

References

Abiru S, Migita K, Maeda Y, et al. "Serum cytokine and soluble cytokine receptor levels in patients with nonalcoholic steatohepatitis." *Liver Int.* 2006; 26:39-45.

Ajmera V, Perito ER, Bass NM, et al. NASH Clinical Research Network. "Novel plasma biomarkers associated with liver disease severity in adults with nonalcoholic fatty liver disease." *Hepatology* 2017; 65:65-77.

Chalasani N, Deeg MA, Crabb DW. Systemic levels of lipid peroxidation and its metabolic and dietary correlates in patients with nonalcoholic steatohepatitis. *Am. J. Gastroenterol.* 2004; 99:1497-502.

Castera L, Friedrich-Rust M and Loomba R. "Noninvasive Assessment of Liver Disease in Patients with Nonalcoholic Fatty Liver Disease." *Gastroenterology.* 2019; 156(5):1264-1281.

Cusi K, Chang Z, Harrison S, et al. "Limited value of plasma cytokeratin-18 as a biomarker for NASH and fibrosis in patients with nonalcoholic fatty liver disease." *J. Hepatol.* 2014; 60(1):167-74.

Feldstein AE, Wieckowska A, Lopez AR, Liu YC, Zein NN, McCullough AJ. "Cytokeratin-18 fragment levels as noninvasive biomarkers for nonalcoholic steatohepatitis: a multicenter validation study." *Hepatology* 2009; 50(4):1072-8.

Hartley JL, Brown RM, Tybulewicz A, et al. "Hyaluronic acid predicts hepatic fibrosis in children with hepatic disease." *J. Pediatr. Gastroenterol. Nutr.* 2006; 43:217-21.

Hui JM, Farrell GC, Kench JG, et al. "High sensitivity C-reactive protein values do not reliably predict the severity of histological changes in NAFLD." *Hepatology* 2004; 39:1458-9.

Hui JM, Hodge A, Farrell GC, et al. "Beyond insulin resistance in NASH: TNFalpha or adiponectin?" *Hepatology* 2004; 40:46-54.

Jarrar MH, Baranova A, Collantes R, et al. "Adipokines and cytokines in nonalcoholic fatty liver disease." *Aliment. Pharmacol. Ther.* 2008; 27:412-21.

Kaneda H, Hashimoto E, Yatsuji S, et al. "Hyaluronic acid levels can predict severe fibrosis and platelet counts can predict cirrhosis in patients with nonalcoholic fatty liver disease." *J. Gastroenterol. Hepatol.* 2006; 21:1458-65.

Musso G, Gambino R, Cassader M, et al. "Meta-analysis natural history of nonalcoholic fatty liver disease (NAFLD) and diagnostic accuracy of non-invasive tests for liver disease severity." *Ann. Med.* 2011; 43:617-49.

Pepe MS, Etzioni R, Feng Z, et al. "Phases of biomarker development for early detection of cancer." *J. Natl. Cancer Inst.* 2001; 93(14):1054-61.

Piperno A, Sampietro M, Pietrangelo A, et al. "Heterogeneity of hemochromatosis in Italy." *Gastroenterology* 1998; 144:996-1002.

Ruiz-Tovar J, Zubiaga L. Validation of biochemical scores for liver steatosis before and 1 year after sleeve gastrectomy. *Surg. Obes. Relat. Dis.* 2019; in press. Doi: 10.1016/j.soard.2019.05.004.

Shen J, Chan HL, Wong GL, et al. "Non-invasive diagnosis of non-alcoholic steatohepatitis by combined serum biomarkers." *J. Hepatol.* 2012; 56:1224-9.

Suzuki A, Angulo P, Lymp J, et al. "Hyaluronic acid, an accurate serum marker for severe hepatic fibrosis in patients with non-alcoholic fatty liver disease." *Liver Int.* 2005; 25:779-86.

Targher G. "Relationship between high-sensitivity C-reactive protein levels and liver histology in subjects with nonalcoholic fatty liver disease." *J. Hepatol.* 2006; 45:879-81.

Tsai E, Lee TP "Diagnosis and Evaluation of Nonalcoholic Fatty Liver Disease/Nonalcoholic Steatohepatitis, Including Noninvasive Biomarkers and Transient Elastography." Clin. Liver Dis. 2018; 22(1):73-92.

Wieckowska A, Papouchado BG, Li Z, et al. "Increased hepatic and circulating interleukin-6 levels in human nonalcoholic steatohepatitis." *Am. J. Gastroenterol.* 2008; 103:1372-9.

Williams AL, Hoofnagle JH. "Ratio of serum aspartate to alanine aminotransferase in chronic hepatitis. Relationship to cirrhosis." *Gastroenterology* 1988; 95:734-9.

Yesilova Z, Yaman H, Oktenli C, et al. Systemic markers of lipid peroxidation and antioxidants in patients with nonalcoholic fatty liver disease. *Am. J. Gastroenterol.* 2005; 100:850-5.

Younossi ZM, Jarrar M, Nugent C, et al." A novel diagnostic biomarker panel for obesity-related nonalcoholic steatohepatitis (NASH)." *Obes. Surg*. 2008; 18:1430-7.

In: Liver Steatosis and Bariatric Surgery ISBN: 978-1-53616-444-2
Editors: Jaime Ruiz-Tovar et al.

Chapter 9

EVOLUTION OF LIVER STEATOSIS AFTER SLEEVE GASTRECTOMY

Ramiro Carbajal Nicho[1,*], MD, Andrei Sarmiento Alarcón[2], MD, Nestor Palacios Bran[1], MD and Jorge Orrego Peche[1], MD

[1]Metabolic and Bariatric Surgeon,
Hospital Edgardo Rebagliati, Lima, Perú
[2]Metabolic and Bariatric Surgeon,
Hospital Santa Rosa, Lima, Perú

ABSTRACT

Obesity is a complex, chronic, progressive, and pandemic disease directly associated with the development of NAFLD (NonAlcoholic Fatty Liver Disease), which is considered the commonest liver disease worldwide. In addition, NAFLD is recognized as a condition that may progress to end-stage liver disease like cirrhosis and/or hepatocellular

---

* Corresponding Author's Email: ramiro.carbajal@gmail.com.

carcinoma, bariatric surgery provides improvement or even histological resolution of NAFLD and NASH (NonAlcoholic SteatoHepatitis).

To date, sleeve gastrectomy is the most commonly performed bariatric procedure worldwide, it has demonstrated acceptable and durable weight loss as well as improve NAFLD and NASH.

Keywords: NAFLD, sleeve gastrectomy, liver steatosis

INTRODUCTION

Nonalcoholic fatty liver disease (NAFLD) is the most important cause of liver disease worldwide that is recognized as the liver component of metabolic syndrome [1, 2]. In addition, the experts suggested that NASH may soon become the most common indication for liver transplantation [3].

The estimated prevalence of non-alcoholic fatty liver disease worldwide is approximately 25% and is present in roughly 95% of patients who undergo bariatric surgery [4, 1]. Moreover, the prevalence of NAFLD patients with type 2 diabetes is elevated with a prevalence rate estimated up to 70% [5]. Furthermore, the prevalence of NAFLD in patients who meet the criteria for metabolic syndrome rate has been estimated to be about 79% [6].

NAFLD includes a broad clinical spectrum ranging from nonalcoholic fatty liver to nonalcoholic steatohepatitis (NASH), advanced fibrosis, cirrhosis, and finally hepatocellular carcinoma (HCC) (table 1). It is important to emphasize that there is a strong association between NAFLD and obesity, insulin resistance or type 2 diabetes mellitus (T2DM) as well as dyslipidemia, suggests that NAFLD is the hepatic manifestation of the metabolic syndrome, also those patients have an increased mortality compared with the general population, with an increased risk of cardiovascular disease, hepatocellular carcinoma, and cirrhosis [7, 8].

Bariatric surgery achieves an improvement or even complete resolution of NAFLD in morbidly obese patients, these patients could be treated with laparoscopic sleeve gastrectomy preventing progression of NAFLD. The purpose of this chapter is to summarize the recent evidence about the effect of sleeve gastrectomy on liver steatosis.

NAFLD (Nonalcoholic Fatty Liver Disease)

NAFLD is characterized by histological or radiographic evidence of fat accumulation in the liver (hepatic steatosis), with or without associated inflammation or fibrosis (steatohepatitis) after the exclusion of other causes of hepatic steatosis, including excessive alcohol consumption (< 20g in women and < 30g in men results in a low risk for the development of alcoholic liver injury) [9, 3].

Table 1. Spectrum of NAFLD

Disease	Subclassification	Most common concurrent disease
NAFDL*	NAFL	**AFLD-alcoholic fatty liver disease, Drug-induced fatty liver disease, Hepatitis C virus-associated fatty liver (genotype3), others, Haemochromatosis, coeliac disease, wilson´s disease, A/hypo-betalipoproteinemia lipoatrophy, hypopituitarism, hypothyroidism, starvation, parenteral nutrition, inborn errors of metabolism
	Pure steatosis	
	Steatosis and mild lobular inflammation	
	NASH	
	Early NASH: No or mild (F0-F1 fibrosis)	
	Fibrotic NASH: Significant (≥ F2) or advanced (≥ 3 bridging) fibrosis	
	NASH-Cirrhosis (F4)	
	Hepatocelular Carcinoma	

* **Primary NAFLD**: Associated with metabolic risk factors.

** **Secondary NAFLD:** May coexist with primary NAFLD.

AFLD: Alcoholic Fatty Liver Disease.

NAFL is characterized by steatosis of the liver, involving greater than 5% of parenchyma, with no evidence of hepatocyte injury [3].

Currently, Liver biopsy is the gold standard procedure utilizing the NAFLD activity score (NAS) for characterizing the severity of NAFLD and for diagnosing NASH (table 1) [10, 11].

NAFLD "is defined by the presence of steatosis in > 5% of hepatocytes according to histological analysis or by a proton density fat fraction (providing a rough estimation of the volume fraction of fatty material in the liver) > 5.6% assessed by proton magnetic resonance spectroscopy (HMRS) or quantitative fat/water selective magnetic resonance imaging (MRI)" [11].

"NASH is defined histologically by the presence of hepatic steatosis and two additional features: lobular inflammation and hepatocyte injury (ballooning)" [12] (Table 1).

NAFLD AND BARIATRIC SURGERY

Despite the increasing numbers of patients with NAFLD, therapeutic options are still limited. Weight loss is the main goal for patients with NAFLD because can lead to an improvement in liver biochemical tests, liver histology, serum insulin levels, and quality of life [13, 14]. In this context, Musso G et al. [15], reported that the 5% body weight reduction resulted in improvement in hepatic steatosis, whereas > 7% reduction was associated with NAS (NAFLD activity score) improvement.

There are several options to obtain weight loss, for instance, lifestyle modification, exercise, healthy diet. Moreover, weight loss is often problematic for patients to continue the needed lifestyle changes long term [16].

Bariatric surgery is the most effective long-term therapy for obesity and its complications and has shown to induce biochemical and histologic remission of NAFLD, through mechanisms of action that are both weight loss-dependent and weight loss-independent [17].

The exact mechanisms that lead to an improvement in NAFLD following bariatric surgery are not completely understood. Since Roux-en-Y gastric bypass (RYGB) is the second bariatric surgical procedure most performed worldwide, it is also the one from which the effects on NAFLD have been most studied, although there is also consistent evidence regarding the effects from gastric banding, sleeve gastrectomy and biliopancreatic diversions [18].

The association between NAFLD and type 2 diabetes mellitus (T2DM) has been well established, which could be explained by the insulin-resistance [17-20].

It comes as no surprise that mechanisms by which bariatric surgery improved the features of NAFLD would be related to weight loss, improvements in T2DM, reduced insulin resistance, reduced hyper-lipidemia, and improved components of metabolic syndrome [21, 22].

Other proposed mechanisms would include the altered route of food delivery, which results in changes to the release of the gut and pancreatic hormones, changes in fat distribution, hepatic insulin and free fatty acid metabolism, and changes in adipocytokines and other cytokines [21]. Alterations in hormone secretion affect carbohydrate and lipid metabolism and interfere with hepatic glucose release [21]. In the last few years, recent studies have shown that changes in some gene expression and gut microbiota may also play a pivotal role [23-25].

Yung Lee et al. [26] performed a systematic review and meta-analysis, found that bariatric surgery leads to complete resolution of NAFLD in obese patients. However, some patients develop new or worsened features of NAFLD, Perhaps, the primary limitation of this study is the heterogeneity between included studies.

Roux-en-Y gastric bypass (RYGB) is the most studied bariatric procedure for its effects on NAFLD, a 2019 systematic review found RYGB to have the greatest impact on NAFLD histology among all bariatric procedures and even suggests that bariatric surgery should be considered as a treatment of NAFLD [27, 28].

Effects of RYGB is discussed in detail in another chapter, in this chapter we will discuss the role of sleeve gastrectomy on NAFLD. At the time of writing this chapter the optimal bariatric procedure for patients with obesity and concomitant NAFLD remains to be defined.

SLEEVE GASTRETOMY AND LIVER STEATOSIS

Currently, laparoscopic sleeve gastrectomy (LSG) is the most common performed bariatric procedure worldwide. LSG is considered to be safe and effective bariatric surgery with durable weight loss. In a recent study, was found that there were no statistically significant differences between sleeve gastrectomy and gastric bypass for weight loss or even to comorbidities such as of type 2 diabetes remission, dyslipidemia resolution, quality of live improvement, and late morbidity.

On the other hand, compared with sleeve gastrectomy, gastric bypass resulted in better resolution of hypertension, based on antihypertensive medication use [29].

Regarding advantages of LSG are low rate of complications, the short operative time, the absence of foreign material, the lack of gastrointestinal anastomosis and malabsorption, there is no mesenteric defects created eliminating the risk of internal hernia and has feasibility to be converted into multiple other bariatric procedures, but there are some issues to be considered such as weight regain, gastroesophageal reflux disease and Barrett's esophagus [30, 31].

Several publications have shown the improvement of NAFLD after bariatric procedures as RYGB as well as adjustable gastric banding (AGB), biliopancreatic diversion (BPD). However, little is known regarding this topic after LSG.

In a recent study Alsina ME, Ruiz-Tovar J and Bernabeu A [32], found that six months after sleeve gastrectomy, a significant reduction of liver steatosis is observed, as demonstrated by reduction in the percentage of intrahepatocitary lipids and liver volume, determined by MRS (Magnetic Resonance Spectroscopy) and MRI (Magnetic Resonance Imaging). In another study Esquivel et al. [33] it was found that sleeve gastrectomy significantly improves NAFLD after 12 months of follow-up, showing even a total regression in some of the patients without cases of worsening of the disease.

Outcomes on prospective data from 236 Patients, Karcz et al. [34] observed significant improvements in AST, ALT, triglycerides and high-density lipoprotein (HDL) levels one and three years after SG. NASH patients showed significant losses of body weight and amelioration of NASH status.

Algooneh et al. [35] did a retrospective study of 84 patients diagnosed with NAFLD prior to undergoing SG.

The diagnosis of NAFLD was achieved based on ultrasonographic imaging. A total of 47 patients (56%) showed complete resolution of NAFLD postoperatively.

Witigo von Schonfels et al. [36] performed a retrospective comparison of metabolic data before and after bariatric surgery and comparison of sleeve gastrectomy and Roux-Y gastric bypass, found that both surgery methods improved the NAS significantly, there was not differences with regard to histological recovery between gastric bypass and Sleeve Gastrectomy.

As has been noted the weight loss and improvements in obesity-related comorbidities, such as Type 2 Diabetes, insulin resistance, and hypertriglyceridemia, after sleeve gastrectomy plays a significant role in the improvement of NAFLD.

On the other hand, sleeve gastrectomy has been shown to result in increased FGF-19, decreased FGF-21, increased adiponectin, and decreased leptin, amylin, and ghrelin levels; no effect was seen on circulating bile acids, these aspects could improve the metabolic syndrome and thus may help improve NALFD [37].

FINAL CONSIDERATIONS

Until now, there is no established therapy and there are no evidence-based clinical guidelines about the treatment of NAFLD.

Sleeve gastrectomy could be a therapeutic option for appropriate, morbidly obese patients with NALFD and NASH, but more studies are needed to determine the long-term effects. Regarding this point, there have not been any adequate prospective, double-blind, controlled trials to provide the data necessary.

REFERENCES

[1] Younossi, Z. M., Koenig, A. B., Abdelatif, D. et al. Global epidemiology of nonalcoholic fatty liver disease—meta-analytic assessment of prevalence, incidence, and outcomes. *Hepatology,* 2016; 64:73 - 84.

[2] Dassanayake, A. S. Nonalcoholic Fatty Liver Disease: Identifying the Disease Burden in Sri Lanka. *Euroasian J. Hepato-Gastroenterol.,* 2018; 8:69 - 72.

[3] Perumpail, B., Khan, M., Yoo, E., Cholankeril, G., Kim, D., Ahmed, A. Clinical epidemiology and disease burden of nonalcoholic fatty liver disease. *World J. Gastroenterol.,* 2017; 23:8263 - 8276.

[4] Machado, M., Marques-Vidal, P., Cortez-Pinto, H. Hepatic histology in obese patients undergoing bariatric surgery. *J. Hepatol.,* 2006; 45:600 - 606.

[5] Kwok, R., Choi, K. C., Wong, G. L. et al. Screening diabetic patients for non-alcoholic fatty liver disease with controlled attenuation parameter and liver stiffness measurements: A prospective cohort study. *Gut,* 2016; 65:1359 - 68.

[6] Soresi, M., Noto, D., Cefalu, A. B., Martini, S., Vigna, G. B., Fonda, M. et al. Nonalcoholic fatty liver and metabolic syndrome in Italy: results from a multicentric study of the Italian Arteriosclerosis society. *Acta Diabetol.,* 2013; 50:241 - 9.

[7] Puig, J., Blasco, G., Daunis-I-Estadella, J., Loshuertos, E., Codina, J., Cuba, V., Ortiz, R., Xifra, G., Ricart, W., Pedraza, S., Federici, M., Fernández-Real, J. M. Nonalcoholic fatty liver disease and age are strong indicators for atherosclerosis in morbid obesity. *Clin. Endocrinol.,* (Oxf.) 2015; 83:180 - 186.

[8] Zeb, I., Katz, R., Nasir, K., Ding, J., Rezaeian, P., Budoff, M. J. Relation of nonalcoholic fatty liver disease to the metabolic syndrome:

The Multi-Ethnic Study of Atherosclerosis. *J. Cardiovasc.,* 2013; 7:311 - 8.

[9] Chalasani, N., Younossi, Z., Lavine, J. E. et al. The diagnosis and management of nonalcoholic fatty liver disease: practice guidance from the American Association for the Study of Liver Diseases. *Hepatology,* 2017; 67:328 - 357.

[10] Wilkins, T., Tadkod, A., Hepburn, I. et al. Nonalcoholic fatty liver disease:diagnosis and management. *Am. Fam. Physician,* 2013; 88: 35 - 42.

[11] Hjelkrem, M., Stauch, C., Shaw, J., Harrison, S. A. Validation of the non-alcoholic fatty liver disease activity score. *Aliment Pharmacol. Ther.,* 2011; 34: 214 - 218.

[12] Farrell, G. C., Wong, V. W. S., Chitturi, S. NAFLD in Asia – as common and important as in the west. *Nat. Rev. Gastroenterol. Hepatol.,* 2013; 10:307 - 18.

[13] Keating, S. E., Hackett, D. A., George, J., Johnson, N. A. Exercise and non-alcoholic fatty liver disease: a systematic review and meta-analysis. *J. Hepatol.*, 2012; 57:157 - 166.

[14] Vilar-Gomez, E., Martinez-Perez, Y., Calzadilla-Bertot, L. et al. Weight Loss Through Lifestyle Modification Significantly Reduces Features of Nonalcoholic Steatohepatitis. *Gastroenterology,* 2015; 149:367 - 378.

[15] Musso, G., Cassader, M., Rosina, F., Gambino, R. Impact of current treatments on liver disease, glucose metabolism and cardiovascular risk in non-alcoholic fatty liver disease (NAFLD): a systematic review and meta-analysis of randomised trials. *Diabetologia,* 2012; 55:885 - 904.

[16] Sanyal, A. J., Friedman, S. L., McCullough, A. J. et al. Challenges and opportunities in drug and biomarker development for nonalcoholic steatohepatitis: findings and recommendations from an American Association for the Study of Liver Diseases-U.S. Food and Drug Administration Joint Workshop. *Hepatology*, 2015; 61:1392 - 1405.

[17] Lassailly, G., Caiazzo, R., Buob, D., Pigeyre, M., Verkindt, H., Labreuche, J. et al. Bariatric surgery reduces features of nonalcoholic

steatohepatitis in morbidly obese patients. *Gastroenterology,* 2015; 149:379 - 388.

[18] Cazzo, E., Pareja, J. C., Chaim, E. A. Nonalcoholic fatty liver disease and bariatric surgery: a comprehensive review. *Sao Paulo Med. J.,* 2017; 135: 277 - 295.

[19] Gruben, N.; Shiri-Sverdlov, R.; Koonen, D. P. Y.; Hofker, M. H. Nonalcoholic fatty liver disease: A main driver of insulin resistance or a dangerous liaison? Biochim. *Biophys. Acta,* 2014, 1842, 2329 - 2343.

[20] Orlani, G., Giorda, C., Manti, R. et al. The burden of NAFLD and its characteristics in a nationwide population with type 2 diabetes. *J. Diabetes Res.*, 2016; 2016:2931985.

[21] Bugianesi, E., Moscatiello, S., Ciaravella, M. F., Marchesini, G. Insulin resistance in nonalcoholic fatty liver disease. *Curr. Pharm. Des.*, 2010; 16: 1941 - 1951.

[22] Thaler, J. P., Cummings, D. E. Minireview: hormonal and metabolic mechanisms of diabetes remission after gastrointestinal surgery. *Endocrinology*, 2009; 150:2518 - 2525.

[23] Cummings, D. E., Overduin, J., Shannon, M. H. et al. Hormonal mechanisms of weight loss and diabetes resolution after bariatric surgery. *Surg. Obes. Relat. Dis.*, 2005; 1:358 - 368.

[24] Federico, A., Dallio, M., Godos, J., Loguercio, C., Salomone, F. Targeting gut-liver axis for the treatment of nonalcoholic steatohepatitis: translational and clinical evidence. *Transl. Res.,* 2016; 167: 116 - 124.

[25] Wieser, V., Adolph, T. E., Enrich, B., Moser, P., Moschen, A. R., Tilg, H. Weight loss induced by bariatric surgery restores adipose tissue PNPLA3 expression. *Liver Int.,* 2017; 37: 299 - 306.

[26] Lee, Y., Doumouras, A. G., Yu, J. et al. Complete resolution of nonalcoholic fatty liver disease after bariatric surgery: a systematic review and meta-analysis. *Clin. Gastroenterol. Hepatol.,* 2019; 17: 1040 - 1060.

[27] Nickel, F., Tapking, C., Benner, L., Sollors, J. et al. Bariatric Surgery as an Efficient Treatment for Non-Alcoholic Fatty Liver Disease in a

Prospective Study with 1-Year Follow-up: BariScan Study. *Obes. Surg.,* 2018; 28: 1342 - 1350.

[28] Tannous, K. Fakhry, Rahul Mhaskar, Theresa Schwitalla et al. Bariatric surgery improves nonalcoholic fatty liver disease: a contemporary systematic review and meta-analysis, *Surgery for Obesity and Related Diseases*, https://doi.org/10.1016/j.soard.2018.12.002.

[29] Salminen, P., Helmio, M., Ovaska, J., Juuti, A., Leivonen, M., Peromaa-Haavisto, P. et al. Effect of laparoscopic sleeve gastrectomy vs laparoscopic roux-en-Y gastric bypass on weight loss at 5 years among patients with morbid obesity: the SLEEVEPASS randomized clinical trial. *JAMA,* 2018; 319: 241 - 54.

[30] Weight regain following sleeve gastrectomy—a systematic review. Lauti, M., Kularatna, M., Hill, A. G., MacCormick, A. D. *Obes. Surg*., 2016; 26:1326 - 1334.

[31] Sebastianelli, L., Benois, M., Vanbiervliet, G. et al. Systematic Endoscopy 5 Years After Sleeve Gastrectomy Results in a High Rate of Barrett's Esophagus: Results of a Multicenter Study. *Obes. Surg.,* 2019; 29: 1462 - 1469.

[32] Alsina, M. E., Ruiz-Tovar, J., Bernabeu, A. Evolution of Liver Steatosis Quantified by MR Imaging and MR Spectroscopy, in Morbidly Obese Patients Undergoing Sleeve Gastrectomy: Short-Term Outcomes. *Obes. Surg.,* 2017; 27: 1724 - 1728.

[33] Esquivel, C. M., Garcia, M., Armando, L. et al. Laparoscopic Sleeve Gastrectomy Resolves NAFLD: Another Formal Indication for Bariatric Surgery? *Obes. Surg.,* 2018; 28: 4022 - 4033.

[34] Karcz, W. K., Krawczykowski, D., Kuesters, S. et al. Influence of Sleeve Gastrectomy on NASH and Type 2 Diabetes Mellitus. *J. Obes.,* 2011; 2011:765473.

[35] Algooneh, A., Almazeedi, S., Al-Sabah, S., Ahmed, M., Othman, F. Nonalcoholic fatty liver disease resolution following sleeve gastrectomy. *Surg. Endosc.,* 2016; 30:1983 - 1987.

[36] Von Schönfels, W., Beckmann, J. H., Ahrens, M., Hendricks, A., Röcken, C., Szymczak, S., Hampe, J., Schafmayer, C. Histologic

improvement of NAFLD in patients with obesity after bariatric surgery based on standardized NAS (NAFLD activity score). *Surg. Obes. Relat. Dis.*, 2018; 14:1607 - 1616.

[37] Haluzikova, D., Lacinova, Z., Kavalkova, P., Drapalova, J., Krizova, J., Bartlova, M. et al. Laparoscopic sleeve gastrectomy differentially affects serum concentrations of FGF-19 and FGF-21 in morbidly obese subjects. *Obesity, 2013;* 21, 1335 - 1342.

In: Liver Steatosis and Bariatric Surgery ISBN: 978-1-53616-444-2
Editors: Jaime Ruiz-Tovar et al.

Chapter 10

LIVER STEATOSIS AND ROUX-EN-Y GASTRIC BYPASS (RYGB)

Luciano Deluca[1,2,*], MD, Liliana Parasporo[2], MD, Patricio Cal[1,2], MD and Ezequiel Fernández[1,2], MD

[1]Programa de Cirugía Bariátrica, Hospital Churruca, Buenos Aires, Argentina

[2]Centro de Rehabilitación de Cirugía de la Obesidad, Buenos Aires, Argentina

ABSTRACT

Given the known beneficial consequence of weight loss on NASH and the predictable effect of bariatric surgery on weight loss, several studies have explored the potential role of bariatric surgery on the treatment of NASH. To date, RYGB remains the most extensively studied bariatric surgery as a potential NASH therapy.

In this chapter we will review the actual evidence of the effect of RYGB on liver steatosis, NAFLD and NASH.

* Corresponding Author's Email: deluca.churruca@gmail.com.

Keywords: Steatosis, obesity, Roux-en-Y gastric bypass, NASH, fatty liver

INTRODUCTION

Nonalcoholic fatty liver disease (NAFLD) is an important cause of chronic liver failure in individuals without significant alcohol consumption [1]. It is the hepatic component of metabolic syndrome and is associated with the deposition of triglycerides into the hepatocytes. NAFLD includes a spectrum of syndromes ranging from pure steatosis (PS) to nonalcoholic steatohepatitis (NASH) to cirrhosis, which can lead to end-stage liver failure or development of hepatocellular carcinoma. While NASH is a condition with a high potential to progress to cirrhosis, PS appears to follow a more benign course, with little or no progression to further liver damage.

As a result of the increasing prevalence of obesity, diabetes and metabolic syndrome, nonalcoholic fat liver disease (NAFLD) has become one of the most common cause of chronic liver disease worldwide [2]. In 2016, 39% of adults were overweight and 16%, obese [3]. In Argentina 60% of the population is overweight, and 5% is obese [4].

Differentiating patients with fibrosis, moderate fibrosis and severe fibrosis can be trickysome. For NAFLD patients, the Original European Liver Fibrosis test has been proposed. It includes variables such as age, tissue inhibitor of matrix metalloproteinase 1, hyaluronic acid and aminoterminal peptide of pro-collagen II.

A similar scoring system, the Enhanced Liver Fibrosis panel, excludes age and is also reliable [8]. The limitation for the routine use of these scores is the cost and availa*bility of the specific markers.* Diagnosis of advanced fibrosis is, indeed, an additional indication for bariatric surgery. However, the surgical procedure must induce a slow and progressive weight loss. More aggressive bariatric surgeries leading to more dramatic weight loss and malnutrition may worsen underlying liver disease [5]. Patients with fibrosis have a higher risk for cirrhosis, portal hypertension, hepatocarcinoma and death [6, 7].

RISK FACTORS

Insulin Resistance

It is considered a fundamental step in the development of the metabolic syndrome (MS), which can eventually end type 2 diabetes mellitus (T2DM). Both NAFLD and NASH are strongly linked to insulin resistance, and the relationship between MS and NAFLD is fully recognized. Insulin resistance facilitates the accumulation of fat in both abdominal subcutaneous adipose tissue and visceral abdominal adipose tissue, as well as in the liver.

Gender

NAFLD is more common in man than in women (ratio 2,1), apparently explained by the protective effect of estrogen, which also facilitate insulin function. As estrogen protects, androgens exert a potential ne*gative role in aggressive NASH.*

Ethnicity

The risk related to ethnicity has been researched in large multiethnic populations. It is considered that the prevalence of nonalcoholic fatty liver is higher in the *population of hispanic origin.*

Feeding

In obese patients with NAFLD, fat accumulates in the liver abnormally in the form of triglycerides, which are derived from lipolysis of adipose tissue by 60%, de novo lipogenesis by 26%, and by diet in the form of chylomicrons in 15%. In this abnormal deposit, the dietary imbalance between omega-6 and omega-3 fatty acids appears to be a determining factor. Fructose, which is increasingly consumed as an additive in commercial beverages, can alter lipidic metabolism. There is evidence that high fructose consumption triggers an increase in de novo lipogenesis, dyslipidemia, insulin resistance and obesity with central fat deposition. This de novo stimulus to lipogenesis contributes to increased deposits of fat in the pathogenesis of NAFLD.

PATHOGENESIS

NASH is a metabolic disease probably caused by multifaceted disturbances of hepatic lipid homeostasis. The hystpatogenesis of NAFLD is not fully understood. The theory of the two hits is the most accepted up to date. The first hit is the accumulation of fat in the liver, which takes to oxidative stress. The second hit is the development of inflammation (steatohepatitis).

As a result of insulin resistance vacuols of triglycerides are accumulated by the hepatocyte, leading to fatty liver.

Not all the fatty acids that are inside the liver have an exogenous origin because there is also a synthesis of fatty acids from the acetate. These fatty acids undergo transformations that will lead to different substances: Triglycerides Cholesterol Phospholipids Ketone bodies (after mitochondrial oxidation of fatty acids). Triglycerides bind to apoproteins and form lipoproteins, which is how they leave the liver to the blood. When they increase the fatty acids they accumulate in the form of triglycerides.

Mitochondria are essential for fat metabolism and can be a major source of oxidative stress under conditions of sepsis or lipotoxicity that is associated w*ith mitochondrial dysfunction.*

The fatty accumulation causes changes in hepatocyte's mitochondria leading to the production free radicals, oxidative stress and finally an inflammatory response with risk of fibrogenesis.

Free fatty acids can induce some microsomal lipogenasas of cytochromes p-450 with the consequent production of free radicals, which are hepatotoxic, and lead to the induction of inflammation. The inflammatory process occurs in zone 3 or perisinusoidal. Chronic inflammation stimulates the activation of the strained or ITO cells and progenitors cells of the liver that lead to a reaction at the level of the bile duct with subsequent fibrosis and progression to cirrhosis. This occurs because the stellate or ITO cells, during chronic inflammatory process, lose their ability to store lipids and differentiate into cells with the characteristics of myofibroblasts, which synthesize type 1 and type 3 collagen in the perisinusoidal space with the consequently liver fibrosis developement.

DIAGNOSIS

Diagnosis can be performed according to clinical and imaging criteria. However liver biopsy is the gold standard to assess steatosis, inflammatory activity and fibrosis; and make a differential diagnosis with other liver diseases. Biopsy is necessary but it has its limitations and is not risk-free. Timing is still controversial. Progressively, new studies have been developed and incorporated to investigate the degree of steatosis, inflammation and fibrosis. However standard guidelines are still lacking.

Most patients with NASH are asymptomatic, although some may suffer from fatigue, malaise, or right upper quadrant discomfort. Often the only clinical sign is hepatomegaly, which may not present in all patients. Few have cutaneous signs of chronic liver disease, but ascites, splenomegaly, spider angiomas, and palmar erythema suggest underlying cirrhosis with portal hypertension. However, some patients with NASH may have normal aminotransferase levels. Less than one half of individuals have a higher than normal alkaline phosphatase level, which is almost always modest, and a few have elevated serum conjugated bilirubin levels. The serum albumin and prothrombin time are typically norm*al in the absence of cirrhosis.*

Regarding the lipid profile, the prevalence of metabolic syndrome and insulin resistance increase as the liver fat increases. The triglycerides values may be high, as well as VLDL and LDL and HDL values may be decreased.

Fibrosis is not required to histologically diagnose esteatosis liver, its usually macrovesicular that refers to hepatocytes with a single large intrachytoplastic fat drop displacing the *nucleus to the periphery cell.*

The extent of steatosis is assessed using percentage involvement by steatotic hepatocytes in liver parenchyma and reported as mild (5 - 33%), moderate (33 - 66%), and severe (> 66%). There are main histological scoring systems to grade and stage NASH. Grade refers to the amount of necro-inflammatory activity, which include the degree of steatosis, ballooning, and lobular inflammation. Stage refers to the categorization of the extent and location of fibrosis. The ra*nge of stages goes from 0 to 4.*

Stage 0: no fibrosis
Stage 1: perisinusoidal/pericellular fibrosis
Stage 2: periportal fibrosis
Stage 3: bridging fibrosis
Stage 4*:* cirrhosis
Stage 4: cirrhosis

Medical Treatment

To date, weight loss achieved via lifestyle intervention remains the mainstream treatment of NASH. A recent meta-analysis of 8 randomized controlled trials (RCTs) – 4 of which included post-treatment histology-involving 373 patients, showed that although ≥ 5% total weight loss (TWL) improved hepatic steatosis, a ≥ 7% TWL was required to improve NASH. [13].

Despite its benefits, in a recent trial by Vilar-Gomes et al. less than one third was able to achieve significant weight loss of ≥ 5% and less than 10% was able to achieve weight loss of ≥ 10% in this trial [14].

Other potential therapies to treat NASH include vitamin E, thiazolidinediones, glucagon-like pep- tide-1 (GLP-1) agonist, and obeticholic acid. Thus far, the best evidence is for vitamin E in nondiabetic adults with biopsy-proven NASH; and thiazolidinediones in patients with and without diabetes with biopsy-proven NASH.

Other therapies are currently undergoing research [15]. A low calorie diet (LCD) is recommended prior to the surgery. The optimal duration has not been determined but a preoperative 2-week LCD treatment seems sufficient for most patients in order to decrease liver volume and fat [16].

Roux-en-Y Gastric Bypass as a Treatment of NASH

Given the known beneficial consequence of weight loss on NASH and the predictable effect of bariatric surgery on weight loss, several studies have explored the potential role of bariatric surgery on the treatment of NASH. To date, RYGB remains the most extensively studied bariatric surgery as a potential NASH therapy [17].

Typically, RYGBP involves the creation of a a 30-50 mL pouch by stapling across the stomach, and then setting a Roux-en-Y gastrojejunostomy with a 15 mm stoma. The Roux limb is usually from 60 to 100 cm in length and *the alimentary limb 100 to 200*cm.

Silverman et al. in 1995 evaluated liver histology in 91 patients before and at 2 to 61 months after RYGB. Out of 91 patients, 18 had no steatosis at baseline. Among the 73 remaining patients, 65 experienced reduction in steatosis in follow-up biopsies, 5 with minimal steatosis at baseline showed no change, and 3 had increased steatosis. Thirteen out of 91 patients had perisinusoidal fibrosis (PSF) at baseline—3 with bridging fibrosis, 1 with moderate fibrosis, and 9 with slight fibrosis. Following RYGB, PSF resolved in 10 patients, decreased in 1 patient and remained the same in 2 patients. One patient developed PSF after RYGB [18]. Mathurin et al. conducted a 5-year prospective cohort study on 381 patients with severe obesity. Liver biopsies were performed prior to and at 1 and 5 years after bariatric surgery. Gastric banding, biliopancreatic bypass, and RYGB were performed in 214 (56.2%), 87 (22.8%), and 80 (21%) patients, respectively. Compared to baseline, there was a significant improvement in the prevalence and severity of steatosis (frequency from 82 to 37.7%; extent from 37.4 to 16%) and a significant reduction in NAS (total NAS 1.9 to 1). Inflammation remained unchanged, while levels of fibrosis increased at 5 years (fibrosis stage 0.27 to 0.36). Despite this increase, 96% of patients had fibrosis score ≤ 1 suggesting that there was no clinically significant worsening in fibrosis. [19].

Lassailly et al. in 2015 conducted a 1-year prospective cohort study on 109 patients with biopsy-proven NASH and severe obesity. Liver biopsies were performed prior to and at 1 year after bariatric surgery.

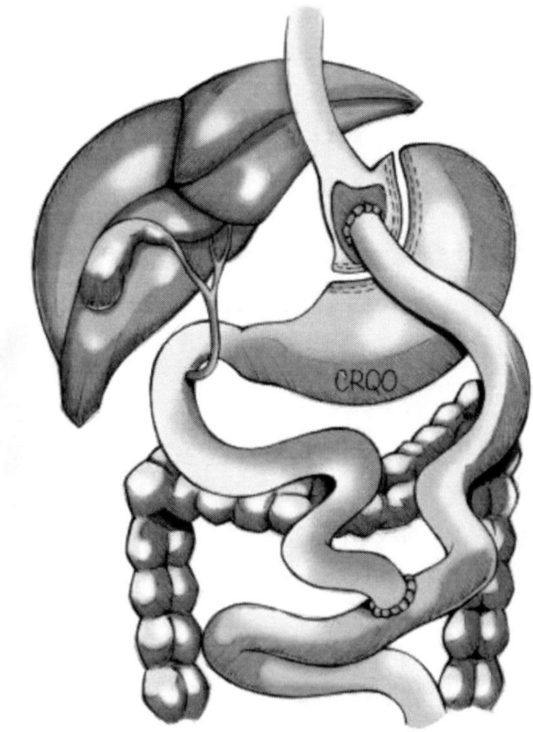

Figure 1. Standard RYGB technique.

Out of 109 patients, 70 (64.2%), 32 (29.4%), 6 (5.5%), and 1 (0.9%) underwent RYGB, gastric banding, sleeve gastrectomy, and biliopancreatic bypass, respectively. One year after surgery, 85% of patients had NASH remission. Compared to baseline, there was a significant reduction in the prevalence of steatosis from 60 to 10%. In contrast to the data from the previous study, fibrosis improved in 34% of the cohort at 1 year after RYGB [20].

A follow-up meta-analysis in 2015 assessed the effect of bariatric surgery on NAFLD liver histology and/or liver biochemistry. The analysis pooled 29 studies and demonstrated a significant reduction in the incidence of all NAFLD histologic features following bariatric surgery: steatosis (16 studies: reduction in the incidence by 50.2%), ballooning (8 studies: 67.7%), lobular inflammation (7 studies: 50.7%), portal inflammation (4 studies: 13.1%), and fibrosis (12 studies: 11.9%) [21].

Histological changes in liver parenchyma can be seen following weight loss of as little as 3 – 5% improving the steatotic burden. Histologic improvement in NASH can be seen at 7% total body weight loss, and decreased fibrosis is seen with further weight loss.

Weight Loss Surgery's (WLS) benefits go beyond slimming down. They are thought to be due to changes in the entero-insulin axis, helping to realign several dysfunctional processes, including insulin resistance, glucose metabolism, and hyperlipidemia [12]. Following RYGB specifically, there are substantial alterations in incretin signaling as part of this process. Increased concentrations of glucagon-like peptide-1 (GLP-1), elevations of gastric inhibitory peptide (GIP), and changes in substances such as peptide YY and oxyntomodulin after RYGB alter enteric signaling pathways. These incretin effects are unique to RYGB and are not seen with non-surgical weight loss. The immediate metabolic effects of RYGB, evidenced by rapid improvements in postoperative hyperglycemia in patients with T2DM, may play a role in biochemical mechanisms by which NAFLD improves. Conversely, the weight loss from the AGB is uniquely due to restrictive effects, while weight loss through VSG comes about primarily through combined restrictive effects and appetite suppression through a decrease in ghrelin. Therefore, improvement of weight-related comorbid conditions tends to be higher with RYGB than with these other commonly offered procedures.

A rare and infrequently event associated with Roux-en-Y gastric bypass is aggressive non- alcoholic steatohepatitis. It is associated with rapid weight loss and/or malnutrition. Roux-en-Y gastric bypass is considered a safe procedure if drastic weight loss is avoided in the postoperative course. The mechanism of liver injury in aggressive steatohepatitis is unknown, but rapid fat mobilization in obese patients may potentially cause oxidative stress to the liver. Further study is needed to determine if there is a genetic predisposition to this form of injury and if antioxidants may protect the liver during rapid weight loss or malnutrition [22].

CONCLUSION

Non-alcoholic fatty liver disease is a known metabolic syndrome's comorbidity. It may potentially lead to fibrosis and cirrhosis. Bariatric surgery may lead to improvement and remission. RYGBP is the most evidence-based treatment. However, special care must be taken on patients with f*aster than average weight loss.*

REFERENCES

[1] McCollough, A. J. Update on non-alcoholic fatty liver disease. *J. Clin. Gastroenterol.,* 2002;34:255 - 62.

[2] Nomura, H., Kashiwagi, S., Hayashi, J., Kajiyama, W., Tani, S., Goto, M. Prevalence of fatty liver in a general population of Okinawa, Japan. *Jpn J. Med.,* 1988;27:142 - 9.

[3] World Health Organization (https://www.who.int/en/news-room/fact-sheets/detail/obesity-and-overweight).

[4] http://www.msal.gob.ar/images/stories/bes/graficos/0000001444cnt-2019- //04_4ta-encuesta-nacional-factores-riesgo.pdf.

[5] Pimentel, S. K., Strobel, R., Gonçalves, C. G., Sakamoto, D. G., Ivano, F. H., Coelho, J. C. Evaluation of the nonalcoholic fat liver disease fibrosis score for patients undergoing bariatric surgery. *Arq. Gastroenterol.,* 2010 Apr.-Jun.; 47(2):170 - 3.

[6] Ratziu, V., Giral, P., Charlotte, F., Bruckert, E., Thibault, V., Theodorou, I., Khalil, L., Turpin, G., Opolon, P., Poynard, T. Liver fibrosis in overweight patients. *Gastroenterology,* 2000; 118: 1117 - 23.

[7] Teli, M. R., James, O. F., Burt, A. D., Bennett, M. K., Day, C. P. The natural history of nonalcoholic fatty liver: a follow-up study. *Hepatology*, 1995;22:1714 - 9.

[8] Guha, I. N., Parkes, J., Roderick, P., Chattopadhyay, D., Cross, R., Harris, S., Kaye, P., Burt, A. D., Ryder, S. D., Aithal, G. P., Day, C. P., Rosenberg, W. M. Noninvasive markers of fibrosis in nonalcoholic fatty liver disease: validating the European Liver Fibrosis Panel and exploring simple markers. *Hepatology,* 2008; 47: 455 - 60.

[9] Verna, E. C., Berk, P. D. Role of fatty acids in the pathogenesis of obesity and fatty liver: impact of bariatric surgery, *Semin. Liver Dis.,* 2008; 28:407 - 426.

[10] Hannah, Jr. W. N., Harrison, S. A. Effect of weight loss, diet, exercise, and bariatric surgery on nonalcoholic fatty liver disease. *Clin. Liver Dis.,* 2016; 20(2):339 - 50. 15. Mason, E. E., Ito, C. Gastric bypass in obesity. *Surg. Clin. North Am.*

[11] Thomas, S., Schauer, P. Bariatric surgery and the gut hormone response. Nutrition in clinical practice: official publication of the American Society for Parenteral and Enteral Nutrition. 2010; 25(2):175 - 82.

[12] Allí, V., Rogers, A. Gastric Bypass and influence on improvement of NAFld. *Curr. Gastroenterol. Rep.,* (2017) 19:25.

[13] Musso, G., Cassader, M., Rosina, F., Gambino, R. Impact of current treatments on liver disease, glucose metabolism and cardiovascular risk in non-alcoholic fatty liver disease (NAFLD): a systematic review and meta-analysis of randomised trials. *Diabetologia,* 2012; 55(4):885 - 904.

[14] Vilar-Gomez, E., Martinez-Perez, Y., Calzadilla-Bertot, L., Torres-Gonzalez, A., Gra-Oramas, B., Gonzalez-Fabian, L., et al. Weight loss through lifestyle modification significantly reduces features of nonalcoholic steatohepatitis. *Gastroenterology,* 2015; 149(2):367 - 78.e5. quiz e14–5.

[15] Chalasani, N., Younossi, Z. The diagnosis and management of non-alcoholic fatty liver disease: *Practice guidance from the American Association for the Study of Liver Diseases*. 2018; 67(1):328 - 57.

[16] Edholm, D., Kullberg, J., Karlson, A., Haenni, A., Ahlstrom, H., Sundbom, M. Changes in liver volume and body composition during 4 weeks of low calorie diet before laparoscopic gastric bypass. *Surgery for Obesity and Related Diseases*, 11 (2015) 602 - 606.

[17] Jirapinyo, P., Thompson, C. Treatment of NASH with gastric bypass. *Current Gastroenterology Reports*, (2018) 20:49.

[18] Silverman, E. M., Sapala, J. A., Appelman, H. D. Regression of hepatic steatosis in morbidly obese persons after gastric bypass. *Am. J. Clin. Pathol.*, 1995; 104(1):23 - 31.

[19] Mathurin, P., Hollebecque, A., Arnalsteen, L., Buob, D., Leteurtre, E., Caiazzo, R., et al. Prospective study of the long-term effects of bariatric surgery on liver injury in patients without advanced disease. *Gastroenterology,* 2009; 137(2):532 - 40.

[20] Lassailly, G., Caiazzo, R., Buob, D., Pigeyre, M., Verkindt, H., Labreuche, J., et al. Bariatric surgery reduces features of nonalcoholic steatohepatitis in morbidly obese patients. *Gastroenterology,* 2015; 149(2):379 - 88. quiz e15–6.

[21] Bower, G., Toma, T., Harling, L., Jiao, L. R., Efthimiou, E., Darzi, A., et al. Bariatric surgery and non-alcoholic fatty liver disease: a systematic review of liver biochemistry and histology. *Obes. Surg.,* 2015; 25(12):2280 - 9.

[22] Mahawar, K. K., Parmar, C., Graham, Y., et al. Monitoring of liver function tests after Roux-en-Y gastric bypass: an examination of evidence base. *Obes. Surg.*, 2016; 26(10):2516 - 22.

In: Liver Steatosis and Bariatric Surgery
ISBN: 978-1-53616-444-2
Editors: Jaime Ruiz-Tovar et al.

Chapter 11

LIVER STEATOSIS REGRESSION AFTER ONE ANASTOMOSIS GASTRIC BYPASS

Luciano Antozzi[1,*]***, MD,***
Miguel Angel Carbajo[2]***, MD, PhD,***
Priscila Antozzi[1]***, MD***
and Carlos Martin Esquivel[3]***, MD, PhD***
[1]Centro de Cirugías Especiales, Bahía Blanca, Argentina
[2]Center of Excellence for the Study
and Treatment of Obesity and Diabetes, Valladolid, Spain
[3]Sanatorio Allende, Córdoba, Argentina

ABSTRACT

The association between *Non Alcoholic Fatty Liver Disease* and obesity has been clearly established, with almost all the obese population suffering some degree of it. Nowadays one third of liver transplants secondary to liver failure are due to NAFLD progression and it is estimated that by 2030 it could become the main cause.

---

* Corresponding Author's Email: lantozzi@gmail.com.

Weight loss can significantly improve NAFLD and bariatric surgery is the most effective long term treatment for obesity and metabolic syndrome.

One anastomosis gastric bypass (OAGB) is a powerful technique with results comparable or superior to more established techniques and it should be considered as part of the armamentarium for treating NAFLD.

Keywords: liver steatosis, non alcoholic fatty liver disease, one anastomosis gastric bypass, cirrhosis

INTRODUCTION

Obesity is a pandemia that co-occurs and interacts with undernutrition and climate change, this constitutes a synergy of epidemics that represent the most serious threat to human health and survival [1].

A large proportion of the obese population suffers metabolic syndrome, type 2 diabetes (T2DM), cardiovascular disease, dyslipidemia and non-alcoholic fatty liver disease (NAFDL). Persistence of this last comorbidity can lead to cirrhosis or hepatocarcinoma.

When liver damage presents with steatosis, steatohepatitis, fibrosis or cirrhosis in patients without alcoholic history, it is considered NAFLD. It affects 10-24% of the general population, but it can rise to 100% when patients are morbidly obese. Besides body fat percentage, central adiposity, hyperinsulinemia and insulin resistance are good predictors of liver dysfunction development [2-8].

Most patients with NAFLD remain asymptomatic or have vague symptoms like fatigue or mild right upper quadrant pain. In stages 3 and 4 of fibrosis, chronic liver disease signs like palmar erythema, telangiectasis or gynecomastia can be found.

During the evaluation of any liver disease, it is important to have initial blood samples of function tests. Most routine biochemical studies have poor correlation with NAFLD. Common blood sample findings are mild to moderate ALT and/or AST elevation. AST/ALT index usually remains under 1 but it rises with fibrosis progression along with gamma-glutamyl transferase. In steatohepatitis, inflammation is present and altered hepatic enzymes are frequently found. Alkaline phosphatase has been found to have statistical association with presence of NAFLD on biopsy [9]. Albumin, prothrombin or bilirubin alteration can indicate liver dysfunction or cirrhosis. In a study with 308 bariatric patients, *highly sensitive C reactive protein* (HSCRP) was found to have utility as an independent predictor of NASH [10].

Ultrasonography has 77% sensitivity and 80% specificity for detecting cirrhosis. For liver steatosis sensitivity rounds 90% with 97% specificity, but it cannot differentiate simple steatosis from steatohepatitis. CT scan and MRI can quantify steatosis and liver volume precisely. Despite imaging studies can detect fatty liver existence, they cannot distinguish hepatic damage severity, this can only be done with liver biopsies, the most precise study for the evaluation of treatment results [11-18].

One third of patients with early stage NASH will progress to fibrosis within 5 to 10 years after the clinical diagnosis has been made when left untreated. Weight loss can produce NAFLD regression, but 90-95% of patients fail to maintain this normal weight with only dietary measures. Bariatric surgery is an important tool to treat obesity comorbidities like NAFLD, being the most commonly performed procedures worldwide Sleeve Gastrectomy (SG) and Roux n Y Gastric Bypass (RYGB). Despite there are concerns about the fast and massive weight loss on liver function, disabsorptive techniques like One Anastomosis Gastric Bypass (OAGB) have demonstrated excellent long-term results. With proper indication and management, this can be a promising treatment for the unstoppable NAFLD rise.

SURGERY AND NAFLD

NAFLD remission or improvement can be related to weight loss, anatomical re-routing, simultaneous remission of comorbidities or by combination of these factors.

There is an established association and coexistence between NAFLD and metabolic comorbidities like insulin resistance (IR), dyslipidemia and T2DM. NAFLD is more severe in diabetic patients and higher rates of fibrosis are found when compared with pre-diabetic or non-diabetic patients [19]. Metabolic effects like improved glucose homeostasis and lipid metabolism and reduced inflammatory activity that would influence NAFLD are observed after bariatric surgery. These effects are due to glucose and lipids metabolism and cannot be entirely explained by weight loss, since they start almost immediately after surgery. Mechanisms of steatosis and ballooning are linked to IR and the long-term evolution may be predicted by early improvement in IR after surgery [20].

Bile acids (BA) act as metabolic modulators and endogenous mediators of energy expenditure and glycolipid metabolism. Enterohepatic circulation is markedly modified when a bilio-pancreatic limb (BPL) without the presence of food is created. The concentration of primary and secondary BA in the portal vein and liver are found significantly elevated due to early reabsorption of the BP limb rather than accelerated transport to the ileum. The length of BPL is of particular importance and affects BA serum rise and they could be responsible for the glycemic control after surgery [21].

Surgery was found to be cost effective, to increase life expectancy, and quality-adjusted survival in patients with all classes of obesity, regardless of fibrosis stage [22]. Many studies have demonstrated significant improvement in histology and beneficial effects on steatosis but, to date, there are no randomized controlled trials showing histological effects of bariatric surgery in NAFLD patients.

Non-invasive methods to evaluate NAFLD changes after surgery, like serologic measurement of metabolic parameters and radiologic tests, are used to generate scores of steatosis or fibrosis. *Fatty liver liver index, NAFLD liver fat score* (steatosis), *Fibrosis 4 score and NAFLD fibrosis score* (fibrosis) are widely validated. Some publications used this method to analyze results but this cannot diagnose NASH [23, 24]. There is still scant data on the durability of NASH remission after surgery proved with biopsy. This can be a major limitation to indicate or conclude which surgery has best results for each patient.

NASH patients are at the highest risk of liver disease progression and dysfunction. Identification of these patients with biopsy and validated histological scoring is important. Bariatric surgery has been found to reduce hepatic fibrosis and necroinflammatory processes, slowing down the process and development of cirrhosis with further complications or death. This natural history of fibrosis or liver failure progression needs to be considered when a cohort of patients is evaluated, because they are most likely to suffer complications or unfavorable progression after surgery.

If cirrhosis is recognized before surgery, patients should be carefully optimized and informed before proceeding to an operation. Even well compensated Child's A patients can safely have surgery. There is no consensus on which bariatric modality is best suited. Access to biliary system and a simpler scenario if a liver transplant is needed are main advantages [25-28].

RESULTS

Bariatric surgery is more effective than medical treatment to achieve sustained weight loss, control insulin resistance, treat T2DM and reduce cardiovascular events. Regarding NAFLD several cohort studies assess the effect of Biliopancreatic Diversion, OAGB, RYGB, Laparoscopic Adjustable Gastric Band (LAGB) or SG. Resolution or improvement of steatosis is the usual findings but there are reports of fibrosis worsening or progression. Transient deterioration of the liver condition mainly occur within the initial postoperative period in which nutritional status and transaminases, cholesterol, albumin or transferrin concentrations can be impaired [29]. LAGB and SG are found less detrimental than techniques that involve disabsorption. Initial liver status has to be evaluated to make proper patient and technique selection.

Numerous studies have pointed out an improvement in steatosis after bariatric surgery after 5 years of follow-up. This long-term evolution can be predicted by early improvement in IR following the surgical procedure. Correlation with weight loss is not linear but Glass et al. described regression in fibrosis when at least 10% of body weight is lost [30]. Luo found 83.7% steatosis resolution and a 21.4% decrease in liver volume at 1 month in 49 patients studied, indistinct of SG or RYGB [31].

In the largest study of BS in NAFLD with more than 500 patients, the effects of RYGB and AGB were compared. Improvement and resolution of steatosis, inflammation and fibrosis were observed after one and five years and the authors did not describe any cases of worsening. Best effects on weight loss and liver histology were achieved in the RYGB patients with greater weight loss and better glucose and lipid metabolism [32].

Another study of 160 patients demonstrated resolution or improvement of steatosis and inflammation in most patients, but 3/37 developed de novo steatosis, 3/114 de novo steatohepatitis and 12/56 de novo fibrosis after surgery, however this result could be affected by the short postoperative period between surgery and biopsy [33].

A recent study found histological NASH in 115 out of 1,489 (7.7%) morbid obese patients. After 109 were submitted to RYGB, LAGB or SG, persistent NASH was more frequent in LAGB than gastric bypass patients (30.4% vs. 7.6%; $p = 0.015$). NASH resolution was diagnosed in 85% of RYGB patients [34].

NAFLD activity score (NAS) higher than 4 is highly predictive of NASH and lower than 3 is highly predictive of its absence [35]. Froylich et al. compared RYGB and SG, they found NAS >4 in 15 patients at the time of surgery and postoperative resolution were achieved in 14. Fibrosis also showed a significant improvement, but 12% of patients in the RYGB arm had worsening fibrosis stage postoperatively [36]. Mathurin et al. using NAS score at 1 and 5 years in 381 bariatric patients found improvement in steatosis and ballooning mainly within the first year that persisted up to 5 years. A lack of significant improvement in inflammation and fibrosis stage worsening at 5 years after surgery was also seen. Refractory IR and insufficient weight loss predicted the persistence of steatosis and ballooning [20].

Some degree of clinical or subclinical hepatic injury within the first year of disabsorptive procedures that generate rapid weight loss has been described [37]. Although progression to cirrhosis or liver failure is rare, there are patients that even required liver transplantation after BPD or Scopinaro [38-40].

A transient elevation in transaminases 6 months after BPD was published in a study of 697 patients, these parameters normalized after 12 months [41]. Biopsies found significant reduction of steatosis and NASH grade as well, confirming low detrimental effects of BPD [42].

Baltasar in a study of 470 patients reported that 10 (2.12%) had hepatic dysfunction not related to viral hepatitis or biliary ductal disease after BPD [43]. Ten years later another publication from the same author reported 1.2% liver disfunction and 0.2% liver failure in a series of 929 patients with the same operation [44].

Giannini et al. investigated the safety of BPD in 56 compensated NAFLD patients at 5 years. Of the patients with baseline NAS score 0-2, it remained unchanged after surgery in 76% of the cases and 24% became indeterminate. Of baseline indeterminate NAS patients, 56% remained unchanged, 41% improved and 3% worsened. Among 8 patients with F3-F4 one remained unchanged, 2 improved to F0-F2 and 5 became indeterminate. None of the patients in this series developed liver related complications. They concluded that liver damage does not seem to be a contraindication to BPD [37].

Texeira reported a patient with BMI 69 kg/m2 submitted to single anastomosis duodeno-ileal bypass (SADI). He consulted at the third year after poor follow-up compliance with 83% EWL, hypoalbuminemia, ascites and cirrhosis [45]. He was treated conservatively but later required revision to RYGB (unpublished).

In a large retrospective analysis of 2,241 patients, Scopinaro did not find any liver failure after his procedure was performed [46].

With jejunoileal bypass (JIB) pioneered by Payne and DeWind, an association between disabsorption and liver complications was found. The technique was abandoned because, among other aspects, the possibility of developing hepatic fibrosis was found in 45% of patients and cirrhosis in 8% [47]. In a review of 6,319 patients, mortality after JIB was 2.8%. Twenty one percent of the 179 fatal cases occurred within 1 month after surgery.

Only 2.9% of patients showed progression of liver disease. In another review, 10 out of 604 patients (1.7%) died of liver failure [48].

Liver impairment mechanism after disabsorptive procedures remains unclear and some groups suggest to avoid this technique if advanced liver compromise is detected prior to surgery. On the other hand, there is a significant association between metabolic comorbidities remission and NAFLD improvement. Disabsorptive techniques are most efficient in this aspect and it is logical to think that best NAFLD remission would be found after they are performed. Only a few studies evaluated what happens with the metabolic effect of surgery when patients regain weight. With re-emergence of initially controlled T2DM and weight recidivism [49], lessening in the improvement of NAFLD outcomes [50] and liver enzymes rise has been demonstrated [51].

The latest guidelines discussing surgical treatment of NAFLD state that surgery is clearly indicated in patients with NAFLD who also meet the criteria for bariatric surgery, but with no specific statement regarding the choice of the procedure [52-53].

OAGB is among the most efficient bariatric techniques regarding long-term results, not only because of weight loss maintenance but also comorbidities resolution. Despite its relative novelty, this technique will find its place within the therapeutic armamentarium for treating NAFLD.

One Anastomosis Gastric Bypass (OAGB)

In 1997, Dr. Robert Rutledge, during a trauma surgery that required antrectomy and intestinal resection, performed a reconstruction with a single gastro-jejunal anastomosis. This reconstruction led to the mini-gastric bypass (MGB) operation, later applied to treat obesity and related comorbidities being less technically demanding than RYGB. In 2001 Dr. Rutledge made the first presentation of excellent results after 1,274 patients. In 2002, Professor Miguel Carbajo, an experienced bariatric surgeon, performed a modification to avoid potential reflux entitling the surgery as one-anastomosis gastric bypass (OAGB) or BAGUA in Spanish. [54] Some modifications have been described with time, trying to reach the operations *State-of-the-art.*

In April 2018 the *International Federation for the Surgery of Obesity and Metabolic Disorders* (IFSO) has determined that the standard nomenclature when referring to the mini gastric bypass described by Rutledge and the one anastomosis gastric bypass described by Carbajo should be One anastomosis gastric bypass (OAGB) [55]. Technical aspects are described below.

MGB consists of a long gastric pouch starting 2-3 cm. below the *Crow's foot* that extends to the angle of His. A 4-6 cm. wide termino-lateral gastro-jejunal anastomosis is constructed leaving a BPL of 150-200 cm. without measuring the total bowel length. In the super obese, the recommended distance to *Treitz* ligament is about 250 cm, in the elderly less than 150 cm. and in type II diabetics without major obesity about 150 cm. [56]

OAGB consists of an 18-20 cm. gastric pouch, an anti-reflux valve conformed by suturing the BPL to the gastric pouch and a latero-lateral gastro-intestinal anastomosis. The most significant difference between surgeries is total bowel length measurement. Bowel length has been found to be variable and this can be important enough to predispose a patient to malnutrition or others to weight regain when fix BPL length is used. Dr. Tacchino observed that 3% of women and 2% of men have small bowel shorter than 400 cm, and interestingly in opposition 15% of men and 5% of women have it longer than 800 cm. [57] Drs. Carbajo and Tovar found in a 5 years prospective observational study of 300 patients that the common limb/total bowel length ratio, followed by common limb length are the most accurate parameters to predict 5-year postoperative BMI below 25 Kg/m2. An ideal range between 0.40 and 0.43 was established (unpublished). They found less variability in total bowel length than Tacchino, but again a group of patients with the risk of a common limb too short was detected if TBL is not measured.

This topic is of particular importance if a patient has liver disease, since the procedure can be tailored knowing the existence of this comorbidity. Longer common limb is safer in these cases. A disabsorption too powerful can lead to not only lack of regression of the disease, but progression or liver failure. Rapid weight loss can affect the liver function.

OAGB and Liver Disease

In a recent systematic meta-analysis, that included studies in English with more than 100 patients as selection criteria, 35 relevant publications about OAGB and 8 registered clinical trials were found. Of this literature review almost every group performed liver function tests and radiologic liver evaluation with US prior to surgical interventions, but results on this topic are barely described.

Eilenberg published a case series of 10 patients with liver dysfunction after RYGB, OAGB and Distal Gastric Bypass. Unfortunately the number of initial surgeries from which this group resulted in is unknown. Three patients had primary OAGB, 2 were converted OAGB after gastric band, 3 had primary RYGB and 2 had RYGB distalization. Clinical presentation was characterized by an increase in liver enzymes, hepato-splenomegaly, thrombocytopenia, impaired coagulation parameters, hypoalbuminemia, and sarcopenia. At later stages, ascites, pleural effusions, encephalopathy and upper gastrointestinal bleeding. Seven developed steatosis/fibrosis and 3 cirrhosis. Eight patients were successfully treated with nutritional preparation and conversion. One OAGB patient required liver transplantation and one RYGB died of decompensated liver disease prior to conversion [58].

Kruschitz retrospective evaluation of 25 non-diabetic patients who underwent OAGB and 25 RYGB found a transient rise in ALT and AST. De Ritis ratio significantly greater in omega-loop gastric bypass after 12 months and faster reduction of GGT in RYGB were observed. Despite the small sample size and that liver biopsies were not available, this is one of few papers assessing important information on this subject [59].

Spivak published a database analysis of 19,053 patients submitted to SG, 2433 to RYGB and 715 to OAGB. EWL superiority was seen in OAGB. Awareness of liver markers on hepatic condition was raised and authors suggest close follow-up if markers at one year switch from normal to abnormal. The percentage of patients with normal baseline AST/ALT that became abnormal was 10%-11.7% in OAGB patients at the first year after the procedure; ALP levels became abnormal in 15.7%. The percentage of patients who went from abnormal to normal AST, ALT, and GGT was significantly higher and outnumbered that of normal to abnormal patients for all 3 procedures, although the differences were lower in OAGB patients [60].

Carbajo reported a 12 years follow-up retrospective study of a prospective database. Of 1200 consecutive patients T2DM, IR, HT, and sleep apnea either totally resolved or substantially improved within the initial period after OAGB. Remission was also demonstrated in most patients for other metabolic conditions like hyperlipidemia and liver steatosis when the first biochemical tests were ordered at the 3rd postoperative month. At 12 years mean EWL was 70%. Early major complications requiring re-operations occurred in 1.3% (9 bleedings and 3 leaks). Two percent of the patients reported sporadic clinical reflux that was managed conservatively [61].

A study of 3000 patients submitted to OAGB showed, after 15 years, a slight to moderate decrease in the percentage of full remission in patients with T2DM (from 94% to 90%), hypertension (from 98% to 87%) and hyperlipidemia (from 98 to 86%) but sustained complete remission of fatty liver disease [62].

Drs. Kular and Rutledge reported their results in a retrospective review of prospective data on 1,054 consecutive patients. With a follow-up of 84% at 6 years they found 85% EWL, 93.2% diabetes and 99% fatty liver remission [63].

Garg et al. researched the utility of transient elastography to evaluate the effect of bariatric surgery on hepatic steatosis and fibrosis with liver stiffness measurement (LSM) and controlled attenuation parameter (CAP). Of 124 patients, 32 underwent biopsy at one year. They found no difference in changes of hepatic steatosis, lobular inflammation, ballooning, NASH and fibrosis between LSG, RYGB and OAGB. Biopsy results were comparable to LSM and CAP [64].

In December 2017 a total of 101 experts from 39 countries evaluated 55 topics during a consensus statement meeting. Seventy-six experts agreed that OAGB is an acceptable surgical option in suitable even in patients with Child-Pugh class A cirrhosis without portal hypertension (75.25% consent) [65].

OAGB Results

It is now widely acknowledged that OAGB is an efficacious technique for achieving sustained weight loss [66-67]. Complete remission or improvement of T2DM is among the greatest found in BS [68-71] and comparable with more complex surgeries like BPD [72-74].

Lee evaluated T2DM remission at one year in 249 MGB and 157 RYGB patients. Complete remission was achieved in 55.4% of patients in RYGB group and in 81.9% of patients in MGB group at 1 year. At 5 year follow-up, results were still significantly better in MGB group (70.5% vs. 39.4%) [75]. The same author in a double-blind randomized trial that included 60 patients, showed MGB superiority over SG in patients with BMI 25-35 kg/m2 up to 5 years after surgery. A statistically significant difference in HbA1C was reported (6.1 ± 0.7 vs. $7.1 \pm 1.2\%$, $p < 0.05$) [76]. Another prospective, randomized clinical trial by Lee compared 40 RYGB and 40 MGB at 2 years follow-up. There were no statistically significant differences in WL, quality of life or clinical results. The author concludes that MGB is a simpler technique than RYGB with similar efficacy [77].

Wang et al. in a systematic review and meta-analysis examined the results of OAGB and SG. EWL was greater after OAGB at one ($p = 0.005$) and five years ($p < 0.001$). Remission of diabetes was significantly better in OAGB ($p = 0.002$) [78]. Quan et al. revised 16 studies and showed superiority of MGB regarding EWL and T2DM remission over SG (89.1% vs. 76.3%, $p = 0.004$) and RYGB (93.4% vs. 77.6%, $p = 0.006$) [79].

Magoulitis et al. in a systematic review of 10 studies that included 6761 patients found that EWL, T2DM and dyslipidemia remission were significantly superior in OAGB than SG. Anyway authors mention that regarding this topic only a small number of RCT were found and results should be cautiously interpreted. The same group compared clinical outcomes of OAGB and RYGB one year later and again found superiority in EWL at five years and T2DM remission, but not dyslipidemia [80].

A recent prospective randomized clinical trial by Tovar compared 600 patients submitted to SG, RYGB and OAGB at 1, 2 and 5 years. Excess BMI lost at 1 year was 81.7 ± 6.3 in SG, 81.2 ± 5.9 in RYGB and 100.4 ± 6.7% in OAGB. At 2 years 87 ± 7.1 in SG, 87.2 ± 6.7 in RYGB and 104.3 ± 7% in OAGB. Both measurements showed significantly better result of OAGB, and no statistically significant different between SG and RYGB. Five years after surgery the same results were found. Final results were in SG group BMI 30.8 ± 2.2, in RYGB 29.9 ± 2.3 and OAGB 25.1 ± 1.8 ($p < 0.001$). Five year remission of diabetes was 82% for SG, 86.4% for RYGB and 95.7% in OAGB. ($p = 0.027$). Five year remission of DL was 28.6% for SG, 71% for RYGB and 100% in OAGB. ($p = 0.001$) [81].

Alkhalifah in a retrospective analysis of a prospective database compared 1731 MGB, 805 RYGB and 1107 SG. Maximum weight loss was achieved in all patients at 2 years. MGB showed significant and durable WL at 10 years. At 2 and 5 years MGB group had the highest remission rates of T2DM (95.1%) and dyslipidemia (87.7%). SG had similar efficacy in diabetes remission rate to both bypass procedures, but significantly lower values in the treatment of dyslipidemia [82].

Jammu and Sharma compared SG, RYGB and MGB in 1107 patients with 52% follow up at 7 years. In the long-term excess weight loss was >90% after MGB, 72% after RYGB and 53% after SG. T2DM remission was 56.5% in SG, 75.8% in RYGB and 95.1% in MGB. DLP remission was 52.4% in SG, 74.0% in RYGB and 93.3% in MGB. Hypoalbuminemia was maximum in MGB. The authors concluded from the results found that MGB was the procedure of choice for patients compliant in taking supplementation [83].

A RCT comparing efficacy of RYGB and OAGB found 60% complete remission of T2DM in OAGB compared with 38% in RYGB [84].

Complications after OAGB

Complications after OAGB are being continuously studied and mostly reported as infrequent. Mortality and early complications rate have been found comparable to SG and RYGB, but with a favorable trend in late complications rate and re-intervention needs. Publications repeatedly mention the possibility of conservative management before the necessity of a surgical intervention. Bile reflux (0.2-2%) and PCM (0.2-1.2%) are main concerns and primary hepatic related complications are not common [85-87].

Revisional surgery is the third most commonly performed bariatric procedure nowadays because of poor primary surgery outcomes. SG can't be reversed, and revision hasn't shown good results, but it is frequently converted. Indications for SG conversion are weight regain, comorbidities persistence and/or GERD. Usually these patients can have a RYGB, BPD or OAGB. After RYGB failure, it is difficult to find a simple and effective solution. Pouch and/or anastomosis reshaping and limb distalization are complex and not very successful. Transformation to OAGB with BPL distalization can achieve comorbidities resolution and weight loss.

OAGB can be revised, converted or reversed with less technical difficulties than RYGB. The main indications are protein calorie malnutrition (PCM), and intractable reflux. These conditions mostly appear within the first 18 months after surgery and should be properly managed clinically before indicating surgery, since most cases respond. Weight regain can also appear in the medium or long-term after MGB.

PCM is associated with poor alimentary habits or to a common limb too short. The incidence is more frequent in vegetarians, diabetic nephropaty, and liver disease patients. Patients can present with lower limbs edema, fatigue and severe hypoalbuminemia.

A systematic review of 12,807 OAGB patients found low postoperative hypoalbuminemia rates (3.4%) and reported occurrence of PCM in 0-3.8% of patients at 2 years [88].

Khalaj et al. in a study of 189 patients submitted to MGB with 200 cm. BPL had the highest published readmission rate secondary to PCM (7/189, 3.7%). Liver function tests were normal in all patients before surgery and 5/7 had different grades of steatosis in US. High serum transaminases was found in only one patient at a mean period of 11.7 +- 4.5 months but rose in 6/7 during follow-up visits. All patients underwent revisional surgery. Of the seven cases, a patient that expired had a history at baseline of DMTII, HT, grade III fatty liver and failed to progress after gastro-gastrostomy. Common limb length in autopsy was 108 cm [89].

Alkhalifah compared SG, RYGB and MGB. Seventy out of 1,731 MGB patients required revision (4%). Malnutrition was the main cause (43 cases) followed by intolerance, and WR. In RYGB revision rate was higher reaching 5.1% with 41.5% secondary to acute internal herniation, 24.4% for WR and 14.6% for malnutrition. SG revision was highest at 5.2% with 89.6% of the cases secondary to GERD or WR [82].

Jammu and Sharma during their initial experience with a longer BPL >250 cm. had 13.1% of patients with hypoalbuminemia and 3.2% of the cases had to be reversed. This observation changed their approach on limb length supporting a shorter BPL [83].

Motamedi reported a morbidly obese patient who underwent MGB that progressed from a baseline NAS 2/8 to 7/8 nine months after surgery. The case was resolved after gastro-gastrostomy [91].

Finally Robert in a multi-centre, non-inferiority, randomized controlled trial found OAGB to be not inferior to RYGB in terms of weight loss and metabolic outcomes at 2 years. Single adverse events can be interpreted as higher throughout the paper but a detailed reading by Mahawar pointed out that actually there was no significant difference in the proportion of patients with at least one serious adverse event (22% with OAGB vs 19% with RYGB; $p = 0.19$). Early and late complications combined was the same for both procedures [92]. The incidence of malnutrition at 2 years was also not significantly different between the groups (OAGB 10.8% *vs* RYGB 16.7%; $p = 0.34$) [84].

Conclusion

Bariatric surgery improves NAFLD in patients with obesity. Despite there are reports of increased de novo fibrosis, development of cirrhosis or liver function alterations are infrequent with modern surgical techniques. Natural progression of NAFLD in the common metabolic syndrome - obesity scenario, makes the decision of performing surgery quite easy. Which technique to choose is far more complex and depends on patients condition, possibility of follow-up, dietary habits and medical team experience or preferences.

There are not many publications specifically addressing liver impact of OAGB but this chapter summarizes that weight loss and comorbidities resolution are of importance for NAFLD control. OAGB is becoming a mainstream because it is proving to be superior to other procedures in these aspects.

Groups starting to adopt this technique should be properly trained and compromised with follow-up and monitoring of liver function tests. If a proper technique and supplementation/diet are utilized, results are optimal and risks minimized.

References

[1] "The Global Syndemic of Obesity, Undernutrition, and Climate Change" *The Lancet Commission report.* 2019-02 https://doi.org/10.1016/S0140-6736(18)32822-8.

[2] Kissebah A, Vydelingum N, Murray R. "Relation of body fat distribution to metabolic complications of obesity" *J Clin Endocrinol Metab* 1982 Feb; 54(2): 254-60.

[3] Reaven GM. "Syndrome X: 6 years later" *J Intern Med Suppl* 1994; 736: 13– 22.

[4] Kvist A, Chowdhury B, Grangard U. "Total and visceral adipose tissue volumes derived from measurements with computed tomography in

adult men and women: Predictive equations" *Am J Clin Nutr* 1988 Dec; 48(6):1351-61.

[5] Gillum RF. "The association of body fat distribution with hypertension, hypertensive heart disease, coronary heart disease, diabetes and cardiovascular risk factors in men and women aged 18–79 years" *J Chronic Dis* 1987; 40:421–428.

[6] Micciolo R, Bosello O, Ferrari P. " The association of body fat location with hemodynamic and metabolic status in men and women aged 21–60 years" *J Clin Epidemiol* 1991;44:591–608.

[7] Bjorntorp P. "Abdominal obesity and the metabolic syndrome" *Ann Med* 1992 Dec;24(6):465-8.

[8] Johnson D, Prudhomme D, Despres. "Relation of abdominal obesity to hyperinsulinemia and high blood pressure in men." *Int J Obes* 1992 Nov;16(11):881-90.

[9] Cazzo E, Gallo F, Pareja J, Chaim E. "Nonalcoholic Fatty Liver Disease in Morbidly Obese Subjects" Correlation among Histopathologic Findings, Biochemical Features, and Ultrasound Evaluation" *Obes Surg*. 2014 Apr; 24(4): 666–668. doi: 10.1007/s 11695-014-1183-4.

[10] Tan C. H., et al. "HSCRP as surrogate marker in predicting long term effect of bariatric surgery on resolution of non-alcoholic steatohepatitis," *Asian Journal of Surgery* (2018), https://doi.org/10. 1016/j.asjsur.2018.04.010).

[11] Palmentieri B, de Sio I, La Mura V. "The role of bright liver echo pattern on ultrasound B-mode examination in the diagnosis of liver steatosis" Digestive Liver Diseases 2006 Jul;38(7):485-9.

[12] Joseph A, Saverymuttu S, al-Sam S. *"Comparison of liver histology with ultrasonography in assessing diffuse parenchymal liver disease."* Clinical Radiology 1991 Jan;43(1):26-31.

[13] Karcaaltincaba M, Akhan O. "*Imaging of hepatic steatosis and fatty sparing.*" European Journal Radiology 2007 Jan;61(1):33-43.

[14] Joy D, Thava V, Scott B. "Diagnosis of fatty liver disease: is biopsy necessary?" *European Journal Gastroenterology Hepatology* 2003 May;15(5):539-43.

[15] Duman D, Celikel C, Tuney D. "Computed tomography in nonalcoholic fatty liver disease: a useful tool for hepatosteatosis assessment?" *Dig Dis Sci* 2006 Feb;51(2):346-51.

[16] Hussain H, Chenevert T, Londy F. "Hepatic fat fraction: MR imaging for quantitative measurement and display early experience" *Radiology* 2005 Dec; 237(3):1048-55.

[17] Kim S, Lee J, Han J. "Hepatic macrosteatosis: predicting appropriateness of liver donation by using MR imaging- correlation with histopathologic findings" *Radiology* 2006 Jul;240(1):116-29.

[18] Machann J, Thamer C, Schnoedt B. "Hepatic lipid accumulation in healthy subjects: a comparative study using spectral fat-selective MRI and volume-localized 1H-MR spectroscopy" *Magnetic Resonance Medicine* 2006 Apr;55(4):913-7.

[19] Souto, Katia P. et al. "Nonalcoholic fatty liver disease in patients with different baseline glucose status undergoing bariatric surgery: analysis of intra-operative liver biopsies and literature review" *Surgery for Obesity and Related Diseases*, Volume 14, Issue 1, 66 - 73. DOI: https://doi.org/10.1016/j.soard.2017.09.527.

[20] Mathurin P, Pattou F et al. "Prospective Study of the Long-Term Effects of Bariatric Surgery on Liver Injury in Patients Without Advanced Disease" *Gastroenterology* 2009;137:532–540. DOI: https://doi.org/10.1053/j.gastro.2009.04.052.

[21] Ise, I., Tanaka, N., Imoto, H. et al. Obesity Surgery (2019) 29: 1901. DOI https://doi.org/10.1007/s11695-019-03790-y.

[22] Klebanoff, MJ, Corey, KE, Chhatwal, J, Kaplan, LM, Chung, RT, Hur, C. "Bariatric surgery for nonalcoholic steatohepatitis: a clinical and cost-effectiveness analysis" *Hepatology*. 2017; 65(4): 1156- 1164.

[23] Perysinakis, I, Pappis, H.C. & Margaris, E. Obesity Surgery (2019) 29: 1058. https://doi.org/10.1007/s11695-019-03705-x.

[24] Angulo P et al. "*The NAFLD Fibrosis Score: A Noninvasive System That Identifies Liver Fibrosis in Patients with NAFLD*" DOI 10.1002/hep.21496.

[25] Wu R, Ortiz J, Dallal R. "Is bariatric surgery safe in cirrhotics?" *Hepat Mon* 2013; 13: e8536 DOI: 10.5812/ hepatmon.8536.

[26] Shimizu H, Phuong V, Maia M, Kroh M, Chand B, Schauer PR, Brethauer SA. "Bariatric surgery in patients with liver cirrhosis." *Surg Obes Relat Dis* 2013; 9: 1-6 [PMID: 23201210 DOI: 10.1016/ j.soard.2012.07.021.

[27] Rebibo L, Gerin O, Verhaeghe P, Dhahri A, Cosse C, Regimbeau JM. "Laparoscopic sleeve gastrectomy in patients with NASH- related cirrhosis: a case-matched study" *Surg Obes Relat Dis* 2014; 10: 405-410; quiz 565 DOI: 10.1016/ j.soard.2013.09.015.

[28] Takata MC, Campos GM, Ciovica R, Rabl C, Rogers SJ, Cello JP, Ascher NL, Posselt AM. "Laparoscopic bariatric surgery improves candidacy in morbidly obese patients awaiting transplantation" *Surg Obes Relat Dis* 2008; 4: 159-164; discussion 164-165 DOI: 10.1016/ j.soard.2007.12.009.

[29] Laursen T, Hagemann C, Wei C, Kazankov K, Thomsen K, Knop F, Grønbæk H. "Bariatric surgery in patients with non-alcoholic fatty liver disease - from pathophysiology to clinical effects" *World J Hepatol.* Feb 27, 2019; 11(2): 138-149. DOI: 10.4254/wjh.v11.i2. 138.

[30] Glass LM, Dickson RC, Anderson JC, Suriawinata AA, Putra J, Berk BS, et al. "Total body weight loss of >/ = 10% is associated with improved hepatic fibrosis in patients with nonalcoholic steatohepatitis" *Dig Dis Sci* 2015;60(4):1024–30).

[31] Luo, RB, Suzuki, T, Hooker, JC. et al. "How bariatric surgery affects liver volume and fat density in NAFLD patients" *Surg Endosc* (2018) 32: 1675. https://doi.org/10.1007/s00464-017-5846-9.

[32] Caiazzo R, Lassailly G, Leteurtre E, Baud G, Verkindt H, Raverdy V, Buob D, Pigeyre M, Mathurin P, Pattou F. "Roux-en-Y gastric bypass versus adjustable gastric banding to reduce nonalcoholic fatty liver disease: a 5-year controlled longitudinal study." *Ann Surg* 2014; 260: 893-898; discussion 898-899.

[33] Taitano AA, Markow M, Finan JE, Wheeler DE, Gonzalvo JP, Murr MM. "Bariatric surgery improves histological features of nonalcoholic fatty liver disease and liver fibrosis." *J Gastrointest Surg* 2015; 19: 429-436).

[34] Lassailly G, Caiazzo R, Buob D, Pigeyre M, Verkindt H, Labreuche J, Raverdy V, Leteurtre E, Dharancy S, Louvet A, Romon M, Duhamel A, Pattou F, Mathurin P, "Bariatric Surgery Reduces Features of Non-alcoholic Steatohepatitis in Morbidly Obese Patients." *Gastroenterology* (2015), doi: 10.1053/j.gastro.2015. 04.014.
[35] Kleiner DE, Brunt EM, Van Natta M, et al. "Design and validation of a histological scoring system for nonalcoholic fatty liver disease" *Hepatology* 2005;41(6):1313–21.
[36] Froylich, Dvir et al. "Effect of Roux-en-Y gastric bypass and sleeve gastrectomy on nonalcoholic fatty liver disease: a comparative study" *Surgery for Obesity and Related Diseases*, Volume 12, Issue 1, 127 – 131.
[37] Giannini, EG, Coppo, C, Romana, C. et al. "Long-Term Follow-Up Study of Liver-Related Outcome After Bilio-Pancreatic Diversion in Patients with Initial, Significant Liver Damage" *Dig Dis Sci* (2018) 63: 1946. https://doi.org/10.1007/s10620-018-5052-1.
[38] Auclair M, Martel G, Lapointe R. "Successful orthotopic liver transplantation after bilio-pancreatic diversion with duodenal switch" *Surg Obes Relat Dis*. 2013;9(3):e46-8.
[39] Baltasar A et al. "Liver failure and transplantation after duodenal switch" *Surg Obes Relat Dis.* 2014;10(6):e93-6.
[40] Baltasar A, Serra C, Pérez N, Bou R, Bengochea M. "Clinical hepatic impairment after the duodenal switch" *Obes Surg.* 2004;14(1):77-83.
[41] Keshishian, K. Zahriya, EB. Willes, "Duodenal switch has no detrimental effects on hepatic function and improves hepatic steatohepatitis after 6 months" *Obes. Surg*. 15 (2005) 1418–1423.
[42] Papadia, F, GM. Marinari, G. Camerini, GF. Adami, F. Murelli, F. Carlini, C. Stabilini, N. Scopinaro, "Short-term liver function after biliopancreatic diversion" *Obes. Surg*. 13 (2003) 752–755.
[43] Baltasar, C. Serra, N. Pérez, R. Bou, M. Bengochea, "Clinical hepatic impairment after the duodenal switch," *Obes. Surg*. 14 (2004) 77–83.
[44] Baltasar, "Liver failure and transplantation after duodenal switch" *Surg. Obes. Relat. Dis*. 10 (2014) e93–e96.

[45] Kirkpatrick V, Moon R, Teixeira A, Jawad M. "Cirrhosis following single anastomosis duodeno-ileal switch: A case report" *International Journal of Surgery Case Reports* Volume 45, 2018, Pages 130-132.

[46] Scopinaro N, Adami GF, Marinari GM, et al. "Biliopancreatic diversion." *World J Surg*. 1998;22(9):936-46.

[47] Quaade F. "Jejunoileal bypass for morbid obesity: A bibliographic study and a randomized clinical trial" *Surg Clin North Am* 1979; 59: 1055-69.

[48] Marubbio AT, Rucher RD, Schneider PD et al. "The liver in morbid obesity and following bypass surgery for obesity" *Surg Clin North Am* 1979; 59: 1079-93.

[49] DiGiorgi M, Rosen DJ, Choi JJ, et al. "Re-emergence of diabetes after gastric bypass in patients with mid- to long-term follow-up" *Surg Obes Relat Dis*. 2010;6(3):249–53).

[50] Jimenez, LS, Mendonça Chaim, FH, Mendonça Chaim, FD. et al. "Impact of Weight Regain on the Evolution of Non-alcoholic Fatty Liver Disease After Roux-en-Y Gastric Bypass/ a 3-Year Follow-up" *Obesity Surgery* (2018) 28: 3131. https://doi.org/10.1007/s11695-018-3286-9.

[51] Burza MA, Romeo S, Kotronen A, et al. "Long-term effect of bariatric surgery on liver enzymes in the Swedish Obese Subjects (SOS) study" *PLoS One*. 2013;8(3):e60495.

[52] Chalasani N, Younossi Z, Lavine JE, et al. "The diagnosis and management of nonalcoholic fatty liver disease: practice guidance from the American Association for the Study of Liver Diseases" *Hepatology*. 2018;67:328–57.

[53] European Association for the Study of the L, European Association for the Study of D and European Association for the Study of O. "EASL-EASD-EASO clinical practice guidelines for the management of non-alcoholic fatty liver disease" *J Hepatol*. 2016;64: 1388–402).

[54] Deitel M. "History of the MGB and OAGB Operations" *International Journal of Surgery* https://doi.org/10.1016/j.ijsu.2019.04.018.

[55] Brown W. *"Mini Gastric Bypass-One Anastomosis Gastric Bypass (MGB-OAGB)-IFSO Position Statement Obesity Surgery"* 2018, Volume 28, Number 5, Page 1188.

[56] Rutledge R, Kular K, Manchanda N. "The Mini-Gastric Bypass Original Technique" *International Journal of Surgery*, https://doi.org/10.1016/j.ijsu.2018.10.042.

[57] Tacchino RM. "Bowel length: measurement, predictors and impact on bariatric and metabolic surgery." *Surg Obes Relat Dis* 2015; 11:328-334.

[58] Magdalena Eilenberg, Felix B. Langer, Andrea Beer, Michael Trauner, Gerhard Prager, Katharina Staufer "Significant Liver-Related Morbidity after Bariatric Surgery and Its Reversal—a Case Series" *Obesity Surgery* (2018) 28:812–819.

[59] Kruschitz R et al. "The Effect of Roux-en-Y vs. Omega-Loop Gastric Bypass on Liver, Metabolic Parameters, and Weight Loss" *OBES SURG* (2016) 26:2204–2212 DOI 10.1007/s11695-016-2083-6.

[60] Spivak, Hadar et al. "Omega-loop gastric bypass is more effective for weight loss but negatively impacts liver enzymes: A registry-based comprehensive first-year analysis" *Surgery for Obesity and Related Diseases,* Volume 14, Issue 2, 175 – 180.

[61] Carbajo M, Luque-de-León E, M. Jiménez J, Ortiz-de-Solórzano J, Perez-Miranda M, Castro Alija, M. (2016). "Laparoscopic One-Anastomosis Gastric Bypass: Technique, Results, and Long-Term Follow-Up in 1200 Patients" *Obesity Surgery*. 27. 10.1007/s11695-016-2428-1.

[62] Carbajo MA, Luque-de-León E. "Laparoscopic one-anastomosis gastric bypass (OAGB): Outcomes with 3000 patients during 15 years (Conference)" *17th Mediterranean & Middle Eastern Endoscopic Surgery Association (MMESA) Congress*. Isfahan (Iran) - October 25th– 27th, 2017.

[63] Kular K, Manchanda N, Rutledge R. "A 6-Year Experience with 1,054 Mini-Gastric Bypasses—First Study from Indian Subcontinent" *Obesity Surgery* (2014) 24:1430–1435 DOI 10.1007/s11695-014-1220-3.

[64] Harshit Garg, Sandeep Aggarwal, Shalimar, Rajni Yadav, Siddhartha Dattagupta, Lokesh Agarwal and Samagra Agarwal, "Utility of Transient Elastography (FibroScan) and Impact of Bariatric Surgery on Non- Alcoholic Fatty Liver Disease (NAFLD) in Morbidly Obese Patients" *Surgery for Obesity and Related Diseases*, http://dx.doi.org/10.1016/j.soard.2017.09.005.

[65] Mahawar, Jacques Himpens, Scott A. Shikor, Jean-Marc Chevallier, Mufazzal Lakdawala, Maurizio De Luca, Rudolf Weiner, Ali Khammas, Kuldeepak Singh Kular, Mario Musella, Gerhard Prager, Mohammad Khalid Mirza, Miguel Carbajo, Lilian Kow, Wei-Jei Lee, Peter K. Small. "The First Consensus Statement on One Anastomosis/Mini Gastric Bypass (OAGB/MGB) Using a Modified Delphi Approach" *Obesity Surgery* https://doi.org/10.1007/s11695-017-3070-2.

[66] Musella et al. "The laparoscopic mini-gastric bypass: the Italian experience: outcomes from 974 consecutive cases in a multicenter review and comorbidities resolution" *Surg Endosc* (2014) 28:156–163 DOI 10.1007/s00464-013-3141-y.

[67] Bruzzi, Matthieu et al. "Single anastomosis or mini-gastric bypass: long-term results and quality of life after a 5-year follow-up" *Surgery for Obesity and Related Diseases*, Volume 11, Issue 2, 321 – 326.

[68] Guenzi, M., Arman, G., Rau, C. et al. "Remission of type 2 diabetes after omega loop gastric bypass for morbid obesity" *Surg Endosc (2015)* 29: 2669. https://doi.org/10.1007/s00464-014-3987-7.

[69] Kular K et al. "Seven Years of Mini-Gastric Bypass in Type II Diabetes Patients with a Body Mass Index <35 kg/m2" *Obesity Surgery* (2015) DOI 10.1007/s11695-015-1941-y.

[70] Apers, J., Wijkmans, R., Totte, E. et al. "Implementation of mini gastric bypass in the Netherlands: early and midterm results from a high-volume unit" *Surg Endosc* (2018) 32: 3949. https://doi.org/10.1007/s00464-018-6136-x.

[71] Georgiadou, Despoina et al. "Efficacy and safety of laparoscopic mini gastric bypass. A systematic review" *Surgery for Obesity and Related Diseases,* Volume 10, Issue 5, 984 – 991.

[72] Pontiroli AE, Laneri M, Veronelli A, et al. "Biliary pancreatic diversion and laparoscopic adjustable gastric banding in morbid obesity: their long-term effects on metabolic syndrome and on cardiovascular parameters" *Cardiovascular Diabetology*. 2009;8:3.

[73] Larrad-Jiménez Á, Sánchez-Cabezudo Díaz-Guerra C, de Cuadros Borrajo P, et al. "Short, mid and long-term results of biliopancreatic diversion" *Obes Surg*. 2007;17(2):202–10.

[74] Theodore K. Alexandrides, George Skroubis, Fotis Kalfarentzos "Resolution of diabetes mellitus and metabolic syndrome following Roux-en-Y gastric bypass and a variant of bilio-pancreatic diversion in patients with morbid obesity" *Obes Surg*. 2007;17(2):176–84.

[75] Owaid M. Almalki, Wei-Jei Lee, Keong Chong, Kong-Han Ser, Yi-Chih Lee and Shu-Chun Chen. "Laparoscopic gastric bypass for the treatment of type 2 diabetes: A comparison of roux-en-Y versus single anastomosis gastric bypass" *Surgery for Obesity and Related Diseases,* doi:10.1016/j.soard.2017.12.022.

[76] Wei-Jei Lee & Keong Chong & Yu-Hung Lin & Jih-Hua Wei & Shu-Chun Chen "Laparoscopic Sleeve Gastrectomy Versus Single Anastomosis (Mini) Gastric Bypass for the Treatment of Type 2 Diabetes Mellitus: 5-Year Results of a Randomized Trial and Study of Incretin Effect" *Obesity Surgery* (2014) 24:1552–1562 DOI 10.1007/s11695-014-1344-5.

[77] Wei-Jei Lee, Po-Jui Yu, Weu Wang, Tai-Chi Chen, Po-Li Wei, Ming-Te Huang. "Laparoscopic Roux-en-Y versus Mini-Gastric Bypass for the Treatment of Morbid Obesity A Prospective Randomized Controlled Clinical Trial" *Annals of Surgery* Volume 242, Number 1, July 2005.

[78] Wang FG, Yu ZP, Yan WM et al. "Comparison of safety and effectiveness between laparoscopic mini-gastric bypass and laparoscopic sleeve gastrectomy: a meta-analysis and systematic review" *Medicine* 2017 Baltimore 96:e8924.

[79] Quan Y, Huang A, Ye M et a. (2015) "Efficacy of laparoscopic mini gastric bypass for obesity and type 2 diabetes mellitus: a systematic review and meta-analysis" *Gastroenterol Res Pract* 2015:152852.

[80] Magouliotis D, Tasiopoulou V, Tzovaras G. "One-Anastomosis Gastric Bypass Versus Sleeve Gastrectomy for Morbid Obesity: a Systematic Review and Meta-analysis)" *Clinical Obesity* 8, 159–169, June 2018. doi: 10.1111/cob.12246.

[81] Ruiz-Tovar, J, Carbajo, MA, Jimenez, JM. et al. "Long-term follow-up after sleeve gastrectomy versus Roux-en-Y gastric bypass versus one-anastomosis gastric bypass: a prospective randomized comparative study of weight loss and remission of comorbidities" *Surg Endosc* (2019) 33: 401. https://doi.org/10.1007/s00464-018-6307-9.

[82] Alkhalifah, N, Lee, WJ, Hai, TC. et al. "15-year experience of laparoscopic single anastomosis (mini-)gastric bypass: comparison with other bariatric procedures" *Surg Endosc* (2018) 32: 3024. https://doi.org/10.1007/s00464-017-6011-1.

[83] Gurvinder S. Jammu, Rajni Sharma. "A 7-Year Clinical Audit of 1107 Cases Comparing Sleeve Gastrectomy, Roux-En-Y Gastric Bypass, and Mini-Gastric Bypass" *Obesity Surgery* DOI 10.1007/ s11695-015-1869-2.

[84] Robert, Maud et al. "Efficacy and safety of one anastomosis gastric bypass versus Roux-en-Y gastric bypass for obesity (YOMEGA): a multicentre, randomised, open-label, non-inferiority trial" *The Lancet*, Volume 393, Issue 10178, 1299 – 1309.

[85] Chevallier, JM, Arman, GA, Guenzi, M. et al. "One Thousand Single Anastomosis (Omega Loop) Gastric Bypasses to Treat Morbid Obesity in a 7-Year Period: Outcomes Show Few Complications and Good Efficacy" *OBES SURG* (2015) 25: 951. https://doi.org/10.1007/s11695-014-1552-z.

[86] Noun, R, Skaff, J, Riachi, E. et al. "One Thousand Consecutive Mini-Gastric Bypass: Short- and Long-term Outcome" *OBES SURG* (2012) 22: 697. https://doi.org/10.1007/s11695-012-0618-z.

[87] Musella M, Susa A, Manno E, Luca M, Greco F, Raffaelli, M, Stefano E, Milone M, Bianco P, Vilardi A, Damiano I, Segato G, Pedretti L, Giustacchini P, Fico D, Veroux G, Piazza L. (2017). "Complications Following the Mini/One Anastomosis Gastric Bypass (MGB/OAGB):

a Multi-institutional Survey on 2678 Patients with a Mid-term (5 Years) Follow-up" *Obesity surgery*. 27. 10.1007/ s11695-017-2726-2.

[88] Parmar, CD & Mahawar, KK. "One Anastomosis (Mini) Gastric Bypass Is Now an Established Bariatric Procedure: a Systematic Review of 12,807 Patients" *OBES SURG* (2018) 28: 2956. https://doi.org/10.1007/s11695-018-3382-x.

[89] Khalaj, A, Kalantar Motamedi, MA, Mousapour, P. et al. "Protein-Calorie Malnutrition Requiring Revisional Surgery after One-Anastomosis-Mini-Gastric Bypass (OAGB-MGB)/ Case Series from the Tehran Obesity Treatment Study" *OBES SURG* (2019) 29: 1714. https://doi.org/10.1007/s11695-019-03741-7.

[90] Johnson, WH. et al. "Surgical revision of loop ("mini") gastric bypass procedure: multicenter review of complications and conversions to Roux-en-Y gastric bypass" *Surgery for Obesity and Related Diseases* 3 (2007) 37–41.

[91] Motamedi et al. "Biopsy-proven progressive fatty liver disease nine months post mini-gastric bypass surgery/ A case study" *International Journal of Surgery Case Reports* 39 (2017) 168–171.

[92] Mahawar, KK. "Findings of YOMEGA Trial Need to Be Interpreted with Caution" *OBES SURG* (2019). https://doi.org/10.1007/s11695-019-03856-x.

In: Liver Steatosis and Bariatric Surgery ISBN: 978-1-53616-444-2
Editors: Jaime Ruiz-Tovar et al. © 2019 Nova Science Publishers, Inc.

Chapter 12

SADI-S: Characteristics and Results of a Novel Bariatric Surgery Technique. The Role in NAFLD and NASH

Esteban Martin-Antona, MD,
Oscar Cano-Valderrama, MD, PhD,
Ester Martin Garcia-Almenta, MD, PhD,
Miguel Josa, MD, PhD and Antonio J. Torres, MD, PhD
Department of Surgery, Hospital Clinico San Carlos, Madrid, Spain

Abstract

SADI-S is a new bariatric procedure that basically consists of a sleeve gastrectomy with a one-anastomosis biliopancreatic diversion. SADI-S has been developed to simplify biliopancreatic diversion without modifying its effectiveness.

Long-term results of SADI-S are lacking but the early and medium-term results are encouraging. Natural history of Non-alcoholic fatty liver disease after SADIS has not been previously studied. However, due to the good results on metabolic comorbidities remission after SADIS, we believe that SADI-S will probably provoque a high percentage of remission in Non-alcoholic fatty liver disease.

Herein, we present a study about the relationship between obesity in bariatric surgery patients and genes that are related to hepatocellular carcinoma. In the future, we will study the change on these genes after SADI-S.

Keywords: bariactric surgery, morbid obesity, non-alcoholic fatty liver disease, non-alcoholic steatohepatitis, Single Anastomosis Duodeno Ileal Bypass with Sleeve Gastrectomy, SADIS

Introduction

SADI-S is one of the most recent innovations in bariatric surgery. It represents the continuous research and evolution in this field to find more effective and safer solutions when treating the obesity epidemic and metabolic related diseases. As already occurred with the mini-gastric bypass or one anastomosis gastric bypass, single anastomosis duodenoileal bypass with sleeve gastrectomy is basically a one anastomosis biliopancreatic diversión (BPD)-duodenal switch (DS) procedure and represents another alternative in the armamentarium of the bariatric surgeon. As often occurs with novel procedures, the nomenclature is not yet standardized: it is defined according to different authors as single anastomosis ileal bypass, loop duodenal switch, mini-DS, duodenoenteral omega switch, stomach intestinal pylorus-sparing (SIPS) surgery. With some differences in gastric tube size and intestinal bypass length, the principle is the same: it is less demanding and eliminates the Roux limb and can potentially reduce postoperative complications without losing metabolic effectiveness of the BPD-DS [1, 2].

Malabsorptive bariatric techniques were initially derived from the metabolic outcomes of massive intestinal resection (usually following mesenteric infarction). The first bariatric procedures were the jejuno-ileal bypass and jejuno-colic bypass, techniques which gave good weight loss and improvement/remission of the metabolic conditions accompanying obesity.

Unfortunately, these procedures were associated with severe late nutritional complications that caused them to be abandoned [1, 2]. In an attempt to deal with these nutritional complications, Nicola Scopinaro developed the biliopancreatic diversion with the intention of maintaining malabsorption while avoiding major uncontrolled malabsorption, disruption of the enterohepatic cycle, and the presence of a long blind loop. One of the features of Scopinaro's technique was the concept of "the three limbs": the alimentary limb, biliopancreatic limb and the common channel. Over the years, several different groups have demonstrated different results based on the varying length of these limbs. The Scopinaro procedure was modified in 1988 by Hess et al. into the BPD-DS. It offered two advantages over previous operations: a vertical gastrectomy along the greater curvature to preserve the integrity of the antropyloric region, as well as a modification of the length of the common channel to 100 cm [2].

The major obstacles of BPD-DS are its technical complexity, complication rates, and possibility of long-term nutritional issues. Nevertheless, BPD and BPD-DS are considered among the best options for selected morbidly obese patients with associated diseases.

To simplify such an effective procedure and preserve its principles, the single anastomosis duodenoileal bypass with sleeve gastrectomy (SADI-S) was first described in 2007 by Sánchez-Pernaute and Torres [3]. SADI-S compared with DS eliminates the Roux-en-Y gastric bypass by creating an omega loop, and because of pylorus preservation, bile diversion is unnecessary as the natural barrier remains in place. Preservation of the pylorus provides control of solid stool emptying, reducing the chances of dumping syndrome and assisting in the maintenance of a physiologically based rate of gastric emptying. The immediate benefit is the need for only one anastomosis, thus saving operative time and potentially reducing postoperative complications. Moreover, since it does not require a mesenteric opening, there is a reduced risk of internal hernia. SADI-S is a solution to determining a decrease in the postoperative and nutritional effects of BPD-DS while maintaining weight and metabolic benefits linked to fundus resection, pylorus preservation, duodenal exclusion, ileal brake effect, and fat malabsorption [2].

It also represents a valid option for revisional surgery after failed sleeve gastrectomy (SG). With SADI, the malabsorptive component is added to an essentially restrictive procedure, as the DS is the natural complement to SG for improving weight loss outcomes and sustainability. Furthermore, it is easier for the surgeon to perform a oneloop duodeno-ileal bypass in "virgin territory." Futhermore, when there is evidence of dilation of the sleeve construction, SADI may also be performed with a concomitant resleeve gastrectomy [2].

Moreover, SADI-S is a versatile procedure. According to patient characteristics and surgeon preference, it can be performed with a narrow gastric pouch and a long common channel (300 or 350 cm) or simply remain a malabsorptive procedure with a short common channel (200 or 250 cm) and a wider gastric pouch. Initially, Sanchez-Pernaute technique consisted a wide sleeve gastrectomy (54 French intragastric bougie) and a one-loop duodenal switch with a 200 cm common channel. This was based on analysis of outcomes of BPD variants. The SADI-S with a 200 cm efferent limb, carried an 8% incidence of clinical malnutrition, and 4% of our patients had to be re-operated to lengthen the common channel. Although these lengthening procedures were considered to be secondary to poor dietary compliance, after this experience they chose to perform a safer procedure by enlarging the common channel to 250 cm.

Standardization of nomenclature and technique, together with further studies with long-term outcomes, are needed to confirm the safety and efficacy of SADI-S in the routine surgical management of the obese population.

Results of SADI-S. What We Know So Far

Since SADI-S is a novel technique in bariatric surgery, having been first described by Sanchez-Pernaute et al. in 2007, there is still some lack of long-term results. However, the literature published about this topic reinforces the idea that SADI-S is a safe and effective technique with a similar efficacy to BPD-DS in weight loss and control of comorbidities such as hypertension, sleep apnea and type 2 diabetes mellitus. While some of the induced physiologic mechanisms of both techiques are overlapping, it is thought that others are different and still not well understood.

The prevalence of Non-Alcoholic Fatty Liver Disease (NAFLD) is rising and is estimated to have doubled in the last 20 years, with rates between 2-44% in the European population and 42,6-69,5% in patients with type 2 diabetes mellitus. Reports suggest that 87-94% of bariatric patients demonstrate abnormal non-alcoholic liver pathology [4]. We know that bariatric surgery is associated with a significant reduction in the incidence of a number of histological features of NAFLD as steatosis, fibrosis, hepatocyte ballooning and lobular inflammation. Also, surgery is associated with reduction in liver enzyme levels (ALT, AST, ALP and gamma-GT) [4, 5].

The group of Sanchez-Pernaute pioneered this technique and published some interesting results [6]. For example, for diabetic obese patients they found remission of T2 DM in 84% of operated patients. They have also observed a significative effect of the lypidic profile, with 89% normalizing tryglicerides, 65% HDL, 79% LDL and 96% normal total cholesterol. Hypertension remitted in 52% and improved in 44%. Also, hypoalbuminemia was detected in 12%, low vitamin A levels in 53% and high PTH levels in 54%. Moreover, this group has observed that in the mid-term SADI-S is at least as effective as other malabsorptive techniques such as BPD/DS and significatively reduces the four main cardiovascular risk factors to a higher extent than RYGB [7].

Zaveri et al. published in 2018 their mid-term outcomes at 4 years [8]. For 437 patients operated, they observed a complication rate of 7,7%. The T2 DM remission rate was 97,6%, and the EWL% was 85,7+/-27,3%.

Shoar et al. published the most complete systematic review about efficacy and safety in 2017 [9]. It comprehended 12 studies including 581 SADI-S patients, being a primary procedure in 87,4% and a conversion procedure in 12,6%. The EWL% average was 85% at 2 years of follow-up. About co-morbidities, a remission rate was observed in 74,1% for T2 DM; 96,3% for HTN; 68,3% for dyslipemia; 63,3% for sleep apnea and 87,5% for GERD. Proteic malnutrition was observed in 34% of patients.

Moreover, some studies have been published in recent years comparing the results of SADI-S with other techniques of bariatric surgery.

Moon et al. published a retrospective study in 2015 comparing the safety and effectiveness of the single versus double anastomosis duodenal switch [10]. They studied 111 SADI-S and 74 DS, obtaining comparable results in terms of weight loss (44,2% vs 48,4% at 24 months). They also recommended a close nutritional follow-up for both techniques, finding hypovitaminosis D in 40% to 60% of the patients studied.

Other groups as Sessa et al., have compared the effects of glucose tolerance testing between SADI-S and other bariatric procedures [11]. They published in 2019 their conclusions. Not surprisingly, BPD and SADI-S seems to be associated to an improvement of insulin sensitivity and glucose homeostasis. Also, a reduced risk of hyperinsulinemia and hypoglycemia was observed, associated with RYGBP and SG.

Also in 2019, Wang et al. published an interesting study using a mildly obese and diabetic rat model to compare diabetes remission and micronutrient deficiency between SADI-S and RYGBP. They divided 30 rats in three equal groups, performing sham operation, SADI-S and RYGB [12]. The two latter groups achieved almost the same efficacy in caloric restriction and fasting plasma glucose control without excessive weight loss. They also showed comparable effects on insulin sensitivity and β cell function. It was remarkable that only RYGB showed changes in gut hormones and vitamin E deficit. These results suggest that diabetes improvement is reached through overlapping and distinct mechanisms in each technique.

About the different mechanisms of action depending on the surgical techniques, Pereira et al. published a study in 2018 where they compared post-prandial hormone profiles between BPD-DS and SADI-S [13]. Two groups of 9 patients each with no past or current diabetes underwent a liquid mixed-meal tolerance test. It was observed that after SADI-s the post-prandial hormone secretion profile presented increased GLP-1, gucagon and insulin secretion when compared to BPD-DS. The authors think that the higher levels of GLP-1 after SADI-S could be attributed to bile acids interactions across a longer intestinal length (300 cm) than in BPD-DS (100 cm). This could also explain in part the higher insulin secretion. About the glucagon secretion, the mechanisms remain unclear, but it could also be triggered by bile acids stimulation. It is apparent that there are some mechanisms that need further investigation to understand these results.

Finally, it is important to note that even when it is reasonable to expect good results in the evolution of NAFLD/NASH after SADI-S, it has also been described by Kirkpatrick et al. at least one case with liver cirrhosis following SADI-S [14]. It is thought that this could be secondary to bacterial overgrowth, protein malnutrition and mobilization of free fatty acids from adipose tissue that could exceed the capacity of the hepatocytes to metabolize and cause steatosis and oxidative damage. All these mechanisms are not unique after SADI-S and it is important to keep in mind this possibility after surgery.

Analysis of Liver Genetic Alterations in Patients Submitted to SADI-S

NAFLD has been related to hepatocellular carcinoma (HCC) [15]. As a first step to understand how NAFLD can promote HCC and how bariatric surgery and SADI-S can avoid HCC provoqued by NAFLD, we have studied the liver genetic alterations in a cohort of patients submitted to SADI-S [16]. In the future, our aim is to analyze if bariatric surgery is able to reverse these genetic alterations.

Material and Methods

Twenty-six patients who underwent surgery in the Department of Surgery of Hospital Clínico San Carlos in Madrid (Spain) were included in the study. Seven patients were control patients not submited to bariatric surgery and 19 patients had morbid obesity and underwent SADI-S as a bariatric surgery procedure. All patients signed an informed consent before being included in the study.

A liver sample was collected during the surgery in all the patients. Patients were classified according to the histologic severity of NAFLD as normal liver, mild/moderate steatosis, severe steatosis and non-alcoholic steatohepatitis (NASH). All the controls had a normal liver sample, mild/moderate steatosis was diagnosed in 14 patients, severe steatosis in 3 patients and NASH in 2. Due to the low number of patients in the severe steatosis and NASH groups, these patients were excluded and control patients were compared to patients with mild/moderate steatosis.

Liver samples were stored at -80°C. RNA was isolated by spraying 25-30 mg of the sample with NucleoSpin RNA/Protein system (Macherey-Nagel, Oensingen, Switzerland). Complementary DNA (cDNA) was synthesized using 1 μg of RNA. First it was mixed during 5 minutes at 65°C with primer poli dT (Roche, Basel, Switzerland) and dNTP (Invitrogen, Carlsbard, California, USA). Then it was mixed during one hour at 50°C with reverse transcriptase Superscript III RNase H Reverse Transcriptase (Invitrogen, Carlsbard, California, USA), DTT and RNA inhibitor RNAsin (Promega, Madrid, Spain). Finally, to get the quantitative PCR (RT-gPCR) the 799HT Perkin-Elmer Applied Biosystems system was used with Fast Start DNA Master SYBR Green I Kit (Roche, Basel, Switzerland).

To decide which genes would be studied, a pool analysis was performed at the beginning of the study. cDNA of different patients in the same histologic group was mixed. These cDNA were analyzed for 70 genes. Sixteen genes were chosen because the genetic expression was different in the pooled cDNA from controls and patients with NAFLD. Other 32 genes were chosen after reviewing the published information about this issue. Some of the genes that were finally studied were TGF-B, BMP, IGF2, IGF1, IRS, IR recptor, TGF-A, HGF, Met, IL6, TNF, NADPH. NOX2. Alox5, MMP7, MMP9 and alpha-fetoprotein.

Quantitative variables are expressed as mean (QR). Genetic expression in the control and mild/moderate steatosis was compared using Mann-Whitney U test. Results with a $p < 0.05$ were considered statistically significant.

RESULTS

Table 1. Compares the characteristics of patients in the control and mild/moderate steatosis group

	Control	Mild/moderate steatosis	P
Age (years)	44 (32-55)	51 (41-56)	$p > 0.05$
Gender (% female patients)	71%	53%	$p > 0.05$
Weight (kg)	122 (92-144)	126 (105-140)	$p > 0.05$
Body Mass Index (kg/m^2)	42 (35-42)	44 (43-51)	$p > 0.05$
Glucose (mg/dL)	98 (89-172)	125 (100-147)	$p > 0.05$
Cholesterol (mg/dL)	209 (165-237)	185 (164-198)	$p > 0.05$
HDL (mg/dL)	60 (57-63)	48 (41-55)	0.011
LDL (mg/dL)	133 (84-182)	101 (82-126)	$p > 0.05$
Triglycerides (mg/dL)	93 (73-155)	143 (107-179)	$p > 0.05$
AST (IU/L)	16 (12-22)	15 (25-42)	$p > 0.05$
ALT (IU/L)	14 (13-25)	25 (20-30)	0.045
GGT (IU/L)	18 (15-21)	26 (23-50)	$p > 0.05$
FIB4 Score	0.84 (0.39-1.13)	0.81 (0.66-1.15)	$p > 0.05$

DISCUSSION

TGF-B2 gene expression was higher in the steatosis group than in the control group. This finding is interesting, as TGF-B genes have been related to fibrotic changes. In fact, TGF-B1 is known to have a central role in the development of liver fibrosis [17]. Also TGF-B2 is known to be an important fibrotic factor [18]. This increase in TGF-B2 is relatedo to a decrease in its type 1 receptor (TGF-BR1 = ALK5). This finding has also been found in HCC cells [19]. Another change related to TGF-B family is the increase in Inhibin subunit beta A (InhBA). InhBA increase has been found in fibrotic and chirrhotic livers from rats [20].

Follistatin (FST344), which is also related to TGF-B family, is another gene that was found to be increased in patients with mild/moderate steatosis. FST344 has been found to be increased in patients with liver carcinoma and is related to clinical characteristics of bad prognosis and a higher tumoral size in patients with HCC [21-23].

Another interesting finding was the increase of genes that have classically been associated with HCC, such as IGF2 [24] or AFP. Also, genes that have recently been related to HCC, such as AREG and CK18, were increased in patients with mild/moderate esteatosis.

Insulin receptor (IRS2) which has also been related to liver tumors [25] was elevated in the study group. Genes related to metastasis, such as MMP7 and VEGFB were also increased [26].

Table 2. Comparison of genetic expression in control and mild/moderate stestosis group

Genes	p
ADIPOR2	0.028
TNFA	0.05
MMPT	0.046
KRT18	0.045
FST	0.028
TGF-B2	0.03
TGF-BR1	0.038
INHBA	0.044
INSR	0.024
IRS2	0.021
IGF2	0.011
VEGFB	0.029
IRF2	0.039
AFP	0.013
AFM	0.033

Finally, ADIPOR2, the adiponectin receptor gene expression, was also increased. Adiponectin is a cytokine secreted by adipose tissue that regulates glycemic and lipidid metabolism. This protein has been related to metabolic disorders of the liver [27].

Conclusion

In summary, after studying the liver samples from patients submitted to SADI-S with mild or moderate steatosis we have found an increase in the expression of several genes that could be related to HCC development. In the future, we will study if these changes are reversible. Our aim is to collect liver samples after the surgery to analyze if the genetic alterations disappear with the bariatric surgery.

References

[1] Angrisani L. Single Anastomosis Duodenoileal Bypass with Sleeve Gastrectomy. In: Angrisani L. *Updates in Surgery*. Bariatric and Metabolic Surgery. Indications, Complications and Revisional Procedures. Springer-Verlag, 2017: pp 107-115. ISBN 978-88-470-3944-5.

[2] Sánchez-Pernaute A. Single-Anastomosis Duodeno-Ileal Bypass with Sleeve Gastrectomy (SADI-S) Surgery. In: Agrawal S. Obesity, *bariatric and metabolic surgery*. Springer, 2016: pp 463-467. ISBN 978-3-319-04343-2.

[3] Sánchez-Pernaute A, Rubio Herrera MA, Pérez-Aguirre E, et al. Proximal duodenal-ileal end-to-side bypass with sleeve gastrectomy: proposed technique. *Obes. Surg*. 2007; 17:1614-1618.

[4] Bower, G, et al. Bariatric Surgery and Non-Alcoholic Fatty Liver Disease: a Systematic Review of Liver Biochemistry and Histology. *Obes. Surg*. 2015; 25: 2280-2289.

[5] Shouhed, D, et al. The role of bariatric surgery in nonalcoholic fatty liver disease and nonalcoholic steatohepatitis. *Expert Rev. Gastroenterol. Hepatol.* 2017; 11: 797-811.

[6] Sanchez-Pernaute A, et al. Single Anastomosis Duodeno-Ileal Bypass with Sleeve Gastrectomy (SADI-S). One to Three Year Follow-up. *Obes. Surg*. 2010; 20:1720-1726.

[7] Torres A, et al. Cardiovascular risk factors after single anastomosis duodeno-ileal bypass with sleeve gastrectomy (SADI-S): a new effective therapeutic approach? *Curr. Atheroscler. Rep*. 2017; 19:58.

[8] Zaveri H, et al. Mid-term 4-year outcomes with single anastomosis duodenal-ileal bypass with sleeve gastrectomy surgery at a single US center. Zaveri, H, et al. *Obesity Surgery* 2018; 28: 3062-3072.

[9] Shoar S, et al. Single Anastomosis Duodeno-Ileal Switch (SADI-S): a systematic review of efficacy and safety. *Obes. Surg*. 2017; 27: 3110-3117.

[10] Moon RC, et al. Safety and effectiveness of single- versus double-anastomosis duodenal switch at a single institution. *Surg. Obes. Relat. Dis*. 2019; 15: 245-252.

[11] Sessa L, et al. Effect of single anastomosis duodenal-ileal bypass with sleeve gastrectomy on glucose tolerance test: comparison with other bariatric procedures. *Surg. Obes. Relat. Dis*. 2019; in press. doi: 10.1016/j.soard.2019.04.013.

[12] Wang T, et al. Comparison of diabetes remission and micronutrient deficiency in a mildly obese diabetic rat model undergoing SADI-S versus RYGB. *Obes. Surg*. 2019; 29: 1174-84.

[13] Pereira S, et al. Biliopancreatic diversion with duodenal switch (BPD-DS) and single anastomosis duodeno-ileal bypass with sleeve gastrectomy (SADI-S) result in distinct post-prandial hormone profiles. *Int. J. Obes*. 2019; in press. doi: 10.1038/s41366-018-0282-z.

[14] Kirkpatrick V, et al. Cirrhosis following single anastomosis duodeno-ileal switch: a case report. *Int. J. Surg. Case Rep*. 2018; 45: 130-132.

[15] Charrez B, Qiao L, Hebbard B. Hepatocellular carcinoma and non-alcoholic steatohepatitis: the state of the play. *World J. Gastroenterol.* 2016; 28: 2494-2502.

[16] Martinez J, Miguel B, Galocha G, et al. La expresion de los genes relacionados con el carcinoma hepatoeclular en pacientes obesos con enfermedad hepatica grasa no alcohólica. [The expression of the genes related to hepatoeclular carcinoma in obese patients with non-alcoholic fatty liver disease] *Cir. Esp*. 2017; 95: 180.

[17] Dooley S, ten Dijke P. TGF-B in progression of liver disease. *Cell Tissue Res.* 2012. 347: 245-256.

[18] Latasa MU, Gil-Puig C, Fernández-Barrena MG, et al. Oral methylthioadenosine administration attenueates fibrosis and chronic liver disease progression in MDR2-/-mice. *PLoS One*. 2010; 5: e15690.

[19] Mu X, Lin S, Yang J, et al. TGF-G signaling is often attenuated during hepatotumorigenesis, but is retained for the malignancy of hepatocellular carcinoma cells. *PLoS One.* 2013; 8: e63436.

[20] Deli A, Kreidl E, Santifaller, et al. Activins and activin antagonists in hepatocellular carcinoma. *World J. Gastroenterol.* 2008; 14: 1699-1709.

[21] Miyahara K, Nouso K, Morimoto Y, et al. Pro-angiogenic cytokines for prediction of outcomes in patients with advanced hepatocellular carcinoma. *Br. J. Cancer.* 2013; 109: 2072-2078.

[22] Tomoda T, Nouso K, Miyahara K, et al. Prognostic impact of serum follistatin in patients with hepatocellular carcinoma. *J. Gastroenterol. Hepatol.* 2013; 28: 1391-1396.

[23] Hedger MP, Kretser DM. The activins and their binding protein, follistatin. Diagnostic and therapeutic targets in inmlamatory disease and fibrosis. *Cytokine Growth Factor Rev.* 2013; 24: 285-295.

[24] Chun YS, Huang M, Rink L, et al. Expression levels of insulin-like growth factors and receptors in hepatocellular carcinoma: a retrospective study. *World J. Surg. Oncol.* 2014; 12: 231.

[25] Chettouh H, Fartoux L, Aoudjehane L, et al. Mitogenic insulin receptor-A is overexpressed in human hepatocellular carcinoma due to EGFR-mediated dysregulation of RNA splicing factors. *Cancer Res.* 2013; 73: 3974-3986.

[26] Kanda M, Nomoto S, Nishikawa Y, et al. Correlations of the expression of Vascular Endothelial Growth Factor B and its isoforms in hepatocellular carcinoma with clino-pathological parameters. *J. Surg. Oncol.* 2008; 98: 190-196.

[27] Silva TE, Colombo G, Schiavon LL, et al. Adiponectin: A multitasking player in the field of liver diseases. *Diabetes Metabol.* 2014; 40: 95-107.

In: Liver Steatosis and Bariatric Surgery ISBN: 978-1-53616-444-2
Editors: Jaime Ruiz-Tovar et al.

Chapter 13

SIMULTANEOUS LIVER TRANSPLANTATION AND BARIATRIC SURGERY

David Calatayud*[*], *Eva María Montalvá, Javier Maupoey, Andrea Boscá and Rafael López-Andújar
Division of Hepatobiliopancreatic Surgery and Transplants, Department of Surgery, Hospital Universitari i Politècnic La Fe, Valencia, Spain

ABSTRACT

Combining liver transplant and bariatric surgery at the same time (simultaneous surgery) represents a therapeutical option that can improve, in rapid ways, the basal conditions of NASH and obesity, trying to reduce, in a significant manner, the negative elements attributed to both chronic-inflammatory diseases. Simultaneous surgery can ameliorate some complication intrinsics to transplant surgery, such as rejection, infection, or disease recurrence due to the steatosis. The main disadvantage of simultaneous surgery is the potential to duplicate or potentiate the complications, such as the infections due to leaks in the hepatic or gastric surgical area. Similarly, simultaneous surgery is an aggressive procedure

[*] Corresponding Author's Email: davidcalatayud1975@gmail.com.

where the patients must adapt to important changes that result from the addition of these two major techniques. In fact, patients undergoing liver transplantation have to modify their diet, especially in the first few months following surgery, and at the same time they must learn to use the new therapeutic arsenal that must be maintained life-long in order to avoid rejection of the new organ. Currently, few quality studies can recommend liver transplantation simultaneously to bariatric surgery. In this sense, it is evident that specialists in hepatology and obesity have to work as a team to develop prospective randomized studies and lay the foundations for this therapeutic option.

Keywords: NAFLD, NASH, liver transplantation, cirrhosis, immunosupresion

INTRODUCTION

At present, obesity is a worldwide epidemy. It is defined as a Body Mass Index (BMI) over 30 kg/m^2. In 2005, nearly a quarter of the world's adult population was overweighted (BMI $\geq$ 25 kg/m^2), and approximately 10% of the population was obese [1]. By 2030, it is estimated that the projected burden of obesity will reach 2.16 billion overweighted and 1.12 billion obese individuals, representing 38% and 20% of the world's adult population, respectively [1]. Over the last decades the prevalence has been increasing mostly in Occidental countries, despite growing recognition of its harms and social preventive health programs [2, 3]. In 2014, it was estimated that 35% of men and over 40% of women were obese. By 2030, an estimation suggests more than half of the U.S. population will have a BMI $\geq$ 30 kg/m^2 [1, 2, 4].

In 2018 a consensus document from the First Spanish NAFLD meeting in Seville was published, entitled "Management of non-alcoholic fatty liver disease (NAFLD)". The result was a Clinical practice guideline [5], with some interesting data.

Non-alcoholic fatty liver disease (NAFLD) has become the most frequent cause of chronic liver disease in children and adults. NAFLD is associated with the global epidemy of obesity and metabolic syndrome [6-8], and is a growing cause of advanced liver disease [9, 10]. In the next few years, NAFLD and alcoholic liver disease will become the most prevalent causes of chronic liver disease in our countries.

The prevalence of NAFLD increases in parallel to the prevalence of metabolic syndrome and its components, especially obesity and diabetes mellitus (DM) [11-12].

Among patients with DM, the prevalence of NAFLD is estimated at 40 - 70%, and the prevalence of NASH is around 22% [13].

In the United States, cirrhosis due to non-alcoholic steatohepatitis (NASH) has become the second most common indication for the inclusion in the waiting list, and the third indication for liver transplantation (LT) [14-21]. This same trend is observed in the transplantation registries of other countries.

These patients usually have obesity-related comorbidities with an increased the risk of cardiovascular (CV) disease [14-22].

NASH will become the main indication for liver transplantation in the next decade. In patients with obesity and NAFLD who require transplantation, the indication is typically for decompensated liver disease [7]. Weight loss has been shown to decrease the progression of NAFLD [23]. Weight loss can result in improvements in liver fibrosis and hepatic steatosis [24].

Diet and exercise are the medical weight loss options, but the weight reduction obtained is around 10%.

Bariatric surgery (BS) is not usually performed in patients with cirrhosis; but several studies have shown its safety in patients with non-cirrhotic NAFLD and even NASH [25, 26]. In addition, it has been demonstrated that there is a significant improvement in both fibrosis and steatosis, with regression of fibrosis in 75% of patients and resolution of steatosis in 84% of patients two years after BS [27].

There are different techniques of bariatric surgery, although the most frequently performed are Roux-en-Y gastric bypass (RYGB) and sleeve gastrectomy (SG).

RYGB is considered by many authors the gold standard bariatric surgical procedure, but in comparison with other surgical approaches it has a higher risk of complications [28]. This is important when operating on a population of patients that have an inherently higher morbidity surrounding any surgical intervention. In addition, in the context of LT, the malabsorptive component of RYGB surgery may cause alterations in immunosuppression absorption [29], a situation that does not occur when an SG is performed [30].

The indications for bariatric surgery in the general population are: a BMI $\geq 35kg/m^2$ with obesity-related comorbidities, or a BMI $\geq 40kg/m^2$ [31]. But in the patient with advanced liver disease or who has already undergone a liver transplant, careful consideration is required.

The timing of surgery continues to be a debate: previous to LT, simultaneous with LT, or delayed after LT.

International Liver Transplantation Society (ILTS) and Obesity Consensus

Recently, the International Liver Transplantation Society (ITLS) convened a consensus conference in Venice in 2018, with a global panel of expert hepatologists and transplant surgeons, to develop guidelines on key aspects of NASH in relation to liver transplantation [32].

Some questions were addressed through the critical review of the literature in different working groups to achieve a global consensus through some statements.

Below are the highlights, to focus next on the surgical aspect.

1. **Are the results of liver transplantation different in obese patients?**
   The outcome of LT in patients with NASH-related cirrhosis with or without hepatocellular carcinoma does not differ from that of other liver transplant etiologies as posttransplant survival is similar [14-22, 33-37].

2. **Concerning the natural history of cirrhotic patients on end-stage liver disease, is it different in NASH-related form other etiologies?**
   Patients with NASH-related cirrhosis have increased CV morbidity and mortality compared to patients with cirrhosis of other etiologies. Patients with NASH cirrhosis have lower mortality rates in the compensated state (Child Pugh A) but similar mortality in the decompensated state (Child Pugh B and C) compared to HCV-related cirrhosis [38-43].
3. **Should this increased CV risk be assessed differently in the transplant-listing evaluation?**
   It is described and demonstrated that liver transplant candidates with NASH should be considered at high risk of developing CV events before and after transplantation. The resulting accumulation of CV risk factors should be carefully evaluated by a multidisciplinary team (including a cardiologist and an anesthesiologist at least). The approach to the pre-LT CV assessment will be the same as other etiologies [21-22, 34, 44-53]. There is not enough evidence to recommend a specific CV risk algorithm for NASH patients undergoing LT evaluation. The stress tests should be of interest.
4. **Is it recommended a particular management of comorbidities in the obese candidate for LT?**
   A multidisciplinary approach is always recommended to establish a risk minimization plan, with an appropriate screening for hypertension, diabetes, and dyslipidemia. Medical optimization in NASH-patients with indication for LT is strongly recommended [54-61].
5. **What therapeutic strategies are recommended on the NASH patient in the waiting list for LT?**
   Cardioselective beta-blockers and statins can be considered in patients with Child A-B NASH-related cirrhosis and CV comorbidities [62-67].
   Moderate exercise is recommended with the double objective of losing weight and improving muscle mass. Prehabilitation programs

are increasing in different centers, based on the impact on postoperative recovery and morbimortality [68-72].

6. **Can obesity contraindicate LT?**
   Class I-III obesity alone is not a contraindication for liver transplantation. However, in the presence of medical comorbidities, particularly concurrent diabetes, rigorous patient selection is strongly recommended [73-84].
   Most studies investigating the effect of obesity on posttransplant survival have reported similar posttransplant patient survival across all BMI categories in the absence of concurrent comorbidities.
   But most of these studies have limitations regarding DM-specific data, ascites status for corrected BMI, etc. In addition, most studies are retrospective and/or include an unmatched patient population.
   Optimal control of comorbidities such as obesity and diabetes before transplantation is difficult with medical treatment. Bariatric surgery should be considered as a good tool to achieve these targets.
7. **Bariatric surgery in obese candidate for LT: What type of BS is the most appropriate? When is the optimal timing for bariatric surgery: before, during or after liver transplantation?**
   We will focus this chapter on these questions, with a small review on bariatric surgery.

Bariatric Surgery in the Setting of Liver Transplantation

Bariatric surgery is a safe and effective treatment for severe obesity. There are many randomized controlled trials and cohort studies that demonstrates this [85-90]. BS has a beneficial long-term impact on the risk of mortality [91-93].

After BS, obesity comorbidities such as diabetes and metabolic syndrome, are often improved or resolved [85, 89].

RYGB (Figure 1A) was traditionally considered the "gold standard" surgical approach because of its short-term weight loss results and its long-term durability. Until 2014, 79.5% of bariatric cases were RYGB [94].

Gastric banding (GB) use is decreasing because of its modest weight loss and poor long-term weight loss durability [95].

The use of SG (Figure 1B) has increased significantly due to lower complication rates with comparable weight loss and resolution of obesity associated conditions [96].

Type of Bariatric Surgery

BS in the context of transplantation has some special considerations. We only compared SG to RYGB.

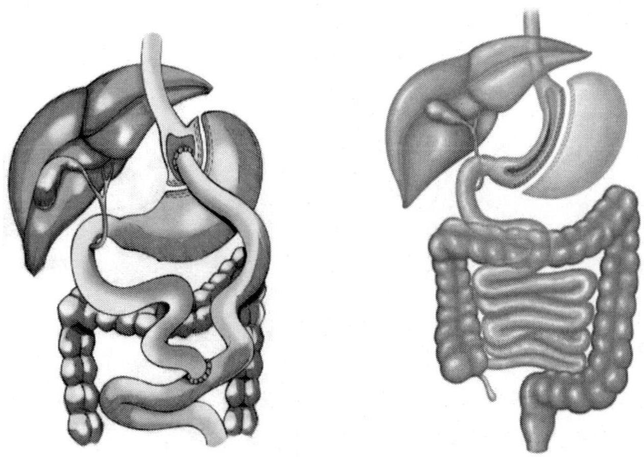

A. Roux-en-Y gastric bypass B. Sleeve gatrectomy

Figure 1. A) Roux-en-Y gastric bypass is a mixed bariatric surgical procedure: restrictive and malabsorptive. B) Sleeve Gatrectomy is a restrictive bariatric surgical procedure, with no malabsorptive component.

Efficacy of GB is limited to case reports. Disadvantages include placement of a foreign body in an immunosuppressed patient with a risk of gastric wall erosion and relative difficulty to endoscopic access if needed.

In many studies, the most common procedure has been SG, up to 100% in some series [97-101]. There are some advantages compared to RYGB:

- technical surgical advantages: minimal additional operative time and no intestinal anastomosis
- postoperative immunosuppression (IS) therapy: it does maintain adequate immunosuppression levels without altering the absorption of medications
- endoscopic procedures: allows endoscopic access to the biliary system for management of posttransplant biliary complications.
- inaccessibility of the gastric remnant if variceal bleeding were to develop when RYGB is performed

Previous reported series have demonstrated steady and gradual EWL% (percentage of excess weight loss) in SG procedure. Takata et al. included both RYGB and SG procedures, SG reported acceptable EWL% (25 - 75%) but lower compared to RYGB [102].

NASH patients constitute a group of increasing LT candidacy. In these patients with metabolic syndrome and other obese-related comorbidities, bariatric prior to transplant or simultaneous LT and BS combined approach might be reasonable in order to have an impact on these risk factors. This should improve both pre and posttransplant outcome.

From Mayo Clinic group in Rochester, one prospective study comparing LT alone to LT-SG demonstrated that the LT + SG group maintained a significantly higher percentage of total body weight loss after 3 years of follow-up. They also had a lower prevalence of hypertension, insulin resistance, and hepatic steatosis and required fewer antihypertensive medications and lipid agents at last follow-up [103].

TIMING OF BARIATRIC SURGERY

Bariatric Surgery before Liver Transplantation

BS in NASH and NAFLD patients has been shown to be effective in both weight loss and improvement in liver pathology [26-27].

In the cirrhotic patients that we find in this group, factors as platelet count, INR, bilirubin, and MELD score can impact on outcomes during BS, with an increased risk and severity of postoperative complications.

Appropriate patient selection may allow pre-LT patients to undergo SG safely. Obesity in LT patients do not increase mortality or worsens graft survival [73]. But, a lower BMI at the time of LT could decrease the risk of wound complications in the short-term and recurrent NASH in the long term [104].

BS before LT seems appropriate for patients with low-MELD score. Particularly with low or no portal hypertension to reduce post-BS morbidity and mortality. This will potentially improve the outcome of LT. Takata and Lin [102, 105] reported significant improvement in metabolic comorbidities, but rates of postoperative complications were significantly higher compared to the general population. But complication rates up to 35% were reported in patients incidentally diagnosed with cirrhosis after BS [106]. This timing could be a good option in low-MELD score patients without portal hypertension.

Simultaneous Liver Transplantation and BS

In 2013, Mayo Clinic published a prospective series of patients who underwent combined LT and SG [107]. In 2018, Mayo Clinic updated their prior experience on long term outcomes [103].

Patients enlisted in the study were all adult patients listed for LT since 2006 with BMI > 35 kg/m^2 (corrected for ascites). These patients were enrolled in an aggressive weight management protocol consisting on dietary education provided by an experienced transplant dietician in subsequent visits until transplantation or achievement of goal weight.

Patients were also evaluated by the same transplant surgeon at the initial and at each subsequent visit to assign a specific weight loss goal (generally BMI < 35 kg/m^2), to further emphasize the long-term benefits of weight loss and to assess progress with weight loss.

Patients were asked to:

1. follow a calorie restricted diet, generally 1200 – 1400 kcal for women and 1400 – 1600 kcal for men,
2. keep an intake record including type, amount and calorie total and bring record to follow-up visits,
3. weigh and record at least once per week and
4. gradually increase activity to 30 – 40 minutes/day, which could be achieved in multiple segments through the day, with walking being the primary recommendation, modified based upon specific patient limitations.

Patients with severe obesity who were unsuccessful with achievement of pretransplant target weight (BMI < 35 kg/m2) who also had a MELD score high enough to allow them to proceed to transplantation underwent a combined liver transplant plus sleeve gastrectomy (LT-SG).

These patients were assessed by the bariatric surgery team and completed the standard bariatric surgery education. All seven LT-SG were performed using deceased donors, with a caval sparing hepatectomy and a duct to duct biliary anastomosis. The SG was performed by an experienced bariatric surgeon following completion of the LT utilizing a 9 mm endoscope placed along the lesser curve of the stomach. A combination of 45-mm 4.8 and 60-mm 3.5 Endo-GIA staple loads were used to resect the antrum and greater curve. Care was taken to leave a small amount of cardia in place in order to avoid injury to the esophagus. The staple line was oversewn using a running 3–0 PDS suture and directly visualized from the lumen of the stomach to ensure hemostasis upon completion, utilizing the previously placed endoscope.

Post-LT management included follow-up visits with the dietician, being counseled on a low-calorie diet plus exercise. Those who underwent combined LT plus SG were seen by the dietician and the bariatric surgery team (surgery, endocrinology and psychology), with the appropriate diet and standard of care in these patients,

In the first report in 2013, obese patients who were unsuccessful with a non-invasive weight loss protocol prior to LT were offered a SG simultaneous with LT (LT-SG) (n = 7). This LT-SG group was compared to a group of obese patients who achieved weight loss via a noninvasive pre-LT weight loss program and underwent LT alone (n = 30). LT-SG group had a MELD of 32 (range 11-40) at time of procedure and 4 out of 7 had NASH as etiology of cirrhosis. Mean operative time was increased by 38 minutes in the LT-SG group and no intraoperative complications were observed. As compared to the non-invasive obesity management, combined LT-SG demonstrated higher resolution of diabetes (100% vs 65,7%) and lower BMI at last follow-up (29 kg/m^2 vs 36 kg/m^2). Two post-operative complications (28.5%) were related to the SG: one staple line leak and one patient with excess weight loss. Heimbach et al. conclude that LT-SG is technically feasible, although not without risk [107].

There are two additional case series/reports of LT-SG from Italy and Israel with similar results: considerable weight loss and no significant perioperative complications [108-109]. But these two articles have two important shortcomings: a short follow-up and a small sample size.

The 2018 publication of the Mayo Clinic provided an update on long-term outcomes for patients who were already enrolled in the 2013 study, plus new recruited patients thereafter [103].

The methodology used with respect to the inclusion criteria was the same as before, but the prevalence of NASH-related cirrhosis is growing over the years. Despite this increasing prevalence, in the US these patients are less likely to be placed on the waitlist, and exhibit higher waitlist mortality, demonstrating that obese patients are disadvantaged on the transplant waiting list [110]. Even that recent reports have noted no difference in patient or graft survival for these patients [73, 75, 111-113]. From the previous Mayo Clinic report in 2013, the aim of this 2018 update was to describe longer-term outcomes, including the dynamics of weight, impact on metabolic outcomes, and quality of life, among these patients after a mean follow-up of 5 ± 2.4 years. They have also provided perioperative and short-term outcomes for the entire cohort of LT + SG patients.

Only patients who were at least 3 years follow-up post transplantation were included in the long-term outcome analysis. Weight and BMI changes were assessed using the percentage of total body weight loss (%TBWL), frequency of a 10% total body weight loss, and the percentage of excess BMI loss (%EBMIL; where BMI = 25 is the normal value). At last follow-up, Adult Treatment Panel (ATP) III criteria was used to assess for metabolic syndrome [114].

It was also updated the evaluation of diabetes (serum determinations of insulin, Homeostasis model assessment index for insulin resistance (HOMA-IR) [115] was calculated and Hemoglobin A1c (HbA1c) was documented [116].

Hepatic steatosis, defined by ultrasound, computed tomography or biopsy, was also evaluated.

And the questionnaire SF-12 version 2 was used to assess quality of life among patients through a phone interview.

There were 74 patients enrolled with 45 undergoing LT alone and 29 undergoing a combined LT + SG. The mean BMI at the time of transplant for the LT-SG group was 47 kg/m^2 (mean weight at LT of 135 kg) with a reduction in BMI to 31 kg/m^2 at last follow-up.

The complication rates were the same as in the previous study. Complications related to SG included one staple line leak, one excess weight loss (stabilized), and two reflux that stabilized at last follow up.

In order to determine the long-term impact of this protocol, only patients with at least 3 years of posttransplant follow-up are included. At three years follow up, LT-SG patients maintained a significantly higher percentage of total body weight loss (%TBWL) when compared to obese LT patients with no combined procedure (LT 3.9 ± 13.3% vs LT-SG 34.8 ± 17.3%; $p < 0.001$) (Table 1).

Table 1. Bariatric parameters and weight dynamics post-surgery

SEBMI	Listing	Transplant	4 months	1 year	2 years	3 years
Weight						
LT	116.4 ± 15.4	95.4 ± 15.0	91.7 ± 16.3	102.2 ± 21.4	111.4 ± 21.1	109.0 ± 18.7
LT + SG	141.6 ± 23.5	128.5 ± 22.8	98.7 ± 18.4	88.6 ± 13.8	90.9 ± 15.3	94.5 ± 25.6
p value	0.002	< 0.001	0.238	0.014	0.003	0.146
%EBWL						
LT	Baseline	17.7 ± 10.5	20.9 ± 11.7	12.1 ± 14.9	4.0 ± 14.5	3.9 ± 13.3
LT + SG		9.1 ± 7.6	29.6 ± 12.3	36.3 ± 12.0	34.4 ± 12.2	34.8 ± 17.3
p value		0.004	0.038	< 0.001	< 0.001	< 0.001
Total body WL > 10%						
LT	Baseline	83.3%	75%	55.6%	29.4%	26,7%
LT + SG		30.8%	84,6%	100%	100%	100%
p value		0.001	0.703	0.004	< 0.001	< 0.001
BMI						
LT	40.0 ± 2.9	32.7 ± 3.7	31.5 ± 5.0	35.1 ± 6.4	38.3 ± 6.8	38.5 ± 6.5
LT + SG	47.8 ± 4.5	43.4 ± 5.6	33.6 ± 6.6	30.3 ± 6.1	31.5 ± 5.7	30.9 ± 13.2
p value	< 0.001	< 0.001	0.324	0.027	0.005	0.130
%EBIL						
LT	Baseline	46.7 ± 28.0	56.4 ± 31.0	32.2 ± 40.4	11.0 ± 39.0	11.0 ± 35.2
LT + SG		19.4 ± 15.3	63.4 ± 27.2	77.0 ± 25.4	72.2 ± 24.1	82.9 ± 70.0
p value		< 0.001	0.455	< 0.001	< 0.001	0.015

Adapted from: Zamora-Valdes D, Watt KD, Todd AK, et al. Long-Term Outcomes of Patients Undergoing Simultaneous Liver Transplantation and Sleeve Gastrectomy. Hepatology. 2018; 68(2): 485–95.

Overall, there was no significant difference observed in the LT alone group between the BMI at listing and the BMI at 3 years (40.06 ± 2.99 vs. 38.53 ± 6.53; difference – 1.52 ± 5.46; P = 0.138) (Figure 2).

In reference to the metabolic syndrome, as shown in Table 2, patients in the LT-SG group had at long term a lower prevalence of hypertension, insulin resistance and hepatic steatosis, and required fewer lipid agents at last follow-up.

In summary, LT-SG group have more effective and more durable weight loss as well as fewer metabolic complications at last follow up when compared to medical weight loss interventions combined with LT.

About the Quality of Life questionnaire, it was a lack of reply, with an overall response rate of 57%. The results of the SF-12 questionnaire showed no significant differences between the two cohorts in any of the categories available.

Bariatric Surgery after Liver Transplantation

This option could be considered since weight loss decreases the risk of recurrent steatosis in the liver graft.

There are few case series with small sample size with a retrospective approach [117-121]. It has been reported a good %EWL and improvement in obesity comorbidities.

Surgeons usually find adhesions and bleeding issues due to reoperation. However, BS after LT is an option for those who develop obesity after transplantation, particularly in patients who were not obese before transplantation.

BS after LT has no impact on comorbidities during the peritransplant period. It has the advantage of a proper selection of patients requiring BS in an elective way, but disadvantages include difficult access to the abdomen and high postoperative morbidity and reoperation rates reported in the literature.

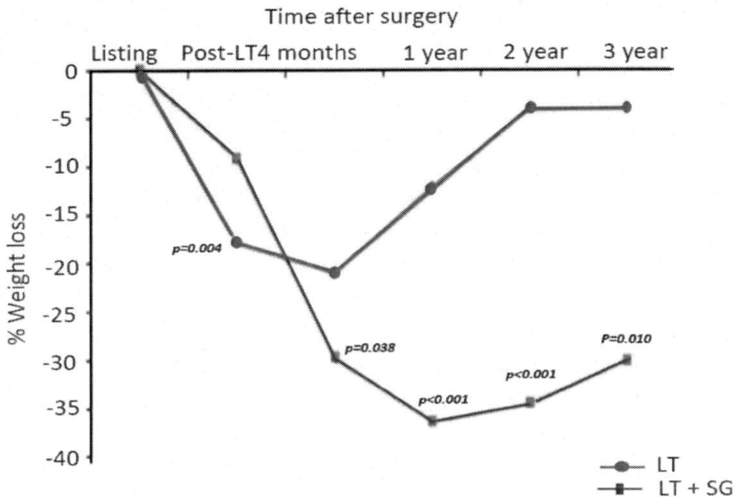

Adapted from: Zamora-Valdes D, Watt KD, Todd AK, et al. Long-Term Outcomes of Patients Undergoing Simultaneous Liver Transplantation and Sleeve Gastrectomy. Hepatology. 2018; 68(2): 485–95.

Figure 2. Percentage of total body weight loss among patients who underwent medical therapy followed by LT and those who underwent LT + SG at listing, transplant, 4 months, 1, 2, and 3 years.

CONCLUSION

NASH is today in 2019 the second major etiology of liver transplantation in the United States, and is expected to become the first in a short time [122]. Obesity comorbidities have a negative impact on graft and patient survival.

Besides, recurrent NAFLD develops in 30 - 60% of patients following LT for NAFLD [123]. This high recurrence rate forces to take preventive measures.

Patients with morbid obesity have more infectious and surgical complications after LT [124-125], and an additional BS may also complicate posttransplantation period.

BS in the peri-transplant period can cause a significant weight loss and a substantial decrease in the incidence of obesity comorbidities, such as diabetes and NASH. This leads to decrease patient morbidity and increase both patient and graft survival.

SG should be considered as a first surgical bariatric option in obese LT patients. SG is a restrictive weight loss procedure that provides durable weight loss results with significant improvement in obesity related comorbidities such as diabetes mellitus, hypertension, and obstructive sleep apnea. In addition, compared to RYGB, there are no changes in IS therapy and the access to the biliary system is maintained.

Bariatric surgery seems to be feasible and effective in morbid obese patients in the setting of liver transplantation, assuming a higher postoperative complication rate.

Bariatric first or concomitant approach might be reasonable for NASH patients who have pre-LT comorbidities including metabolic and CV problems that may complicate the post-transplant period. The optimal type of BS remains unclear, but SG seems to be the preferred approach by most surgeons [97-99, 103].

The optimal time of BS in relation to liver transplantation has not yet been determined.

To date, there are no studies comparing different timing of BS in relation to liver transplantation.

Table 2. Obesity-related comorbidies at last follow-up post-LT

Variable	LT cohort	LT + SG Cohort	p value
Diabetes Mellitus	58.3%	30.8%	0.114
# medication	0.5 ± 0.8	0.3 ± 0.9	0.517
Hypertension	63.9%	23.1%	0.021
# medications	1.0 ± 1.0	0.3 ± 0.7	0.023
Dyslipemia	69.4%	53.8%	0.178
# medications	0.4 ± 0.6	0.1 ± 0.2	0.01
MetS	52.8%	23.1%	0.104
# criteria	2.83 ± 1.0	1.9 ± 0.9	0.008
HS	66.7%	23.1%	0.01

Adapted from: Zamora-Valdes D, Watt KD, Todd AK, et al. Long-Term Outcomes of Patients Undergoing Simultaneous Liver Transplantation and Sleeve Gastrectomy. Hepatology. 2018; 68(2): 485–95.

REFERENCES

[1] Kelly, T; Yang, W; Chen, CS; Reynolds, K; He, J. Global burden of obesity in 2005 and projections to 2030. *Int J Obes.*, 2008, 32(9), 1431-1437. doi:10.1038/ijo.2008.102.

[2] Clinical guidelines on the identification, evaluation, and treatment of overweight and obesity in adults: executive summary. Expert Panel on the Identification, Evaluation, and Treatment of Overweight in Adults. *Am J Clin Nutr.*, 1998, 68(4), 899-917. doi:10.1093/ajcn/68.4.899.

[3] Flegal, KM; Kruszon-Moran, D; Carroll, MD; Fryar, CD; Ogden, CL. Trends in Obesity Among Adults in the United States, 2005 to 2014. *JAMA.*, 2016, 315(21), 2284. doi:10.1001/jama.2016.6458.

[4] Wang, Y; Beydoun, MA; Liang, L; Caballero, B; Kumanyika, SK. Will all Americans become overweight or obese? estimating the progression and cost of the US obesity epidemic. *Obesity (Silver Spring).*, 2008, 16(10), 2323-2330. doi:10.1038/oby.2008.351.

[5] Aller, R; Fernández-Rodríguez, C; lo Iacono, O; et al. Documento de consenso. Manejo de la enfermedad hepática grasa no alcohólica (EHGNA). Guía de práctica clínica. *Gastroenterol Hepatol.*, 2018, 41(5), 328-349. doi:10.1016/j.gastrohep.2017.12.003.

[6] European Association for the Study of the Liver (EASL), European Association for the Study of Diabetes (EASD), European Association for the Study of Obesity (EASO). EASL-EASD-EASO Clinical Practice Guidelines for the management of non-alcoholic fatty liver disease. *J Hepatol.*, 2016, 64(6), 1388-1402. doi:10.1016/j.jhep.2015.11.004.

[7] Rinella, ME. Nonalcoholic Fatty Liver Disease. *JAMA.*, 2015, 313(22), 2263. doi:10.1001/jama.2015.5370.

[8] Loomba, R; Sanyal, AJ. The global NAFLD epidemic. *Nat Rev Gastroenterol Hepatol.*, 2013, 10(11), 686-690. doi:10.1038/nrgastro.2013.171.

[9] Zakhari, S; Li, TK. Determinants of alcohol use and abuse: Impact of quantity and frequency patterns on liver disease. *Hepatology.*, 2007, 46(6), 2032-2039. doi:10.1002/hep.22010.

[10] Rehm, J; Mathers, C; Popova, S; Thavorncharoensap, M; Teerawattananon, Y; Patra, J. Global burden of disease and injury and economic cost attributable to alcohol use and alcohol-use disorders. *Lancet* (London, England)., 2009, 373(9682), 2223-2233. doi:10.1016/S0140-6736(09)60746-7.

[11] Williams, CD; Stengel, J; Asike, MI; et al. Prevalence of nonalcoholic fatty liver disease and nonalcoholic steatohepatitis among a largely middle-aged population utilizing ultrasound and liver biopsy: a prospective study. *Gastroenterology.*, 2011, 140(1), 124-131. doi:10.1053/j.gastro.2010.09.038.

[12] Lazo, M; Clark, J. The Epidemiology of Nonalcoholic Fatty Liver Disease: A Global Perspective. *Semin Liver Dis.*, 2008, 28(04), 339-350. doi:10.1055/s-0028-1091978.

[13] Machado, M; Marques-Vidal, P; Cortez-Pinto, H. Hepatic histology in obese patients undergoing bariatric surgery. *J Hepatol.*, 2006, 45(4), 600-606. doi:10.1016/j.jhep.2006.06.013.

[14] Wang, X; Li, J; Riaz, DR; Shi, G; Liu, C; Dai, Y. Outcomes of liver transplantation for nonalcoholic steatohepatitis: a systematic review and meta-analysis. *Clin Gastroenterol Hepatol.*, 2014, 12(3), 394-402.e1. doi:10.1016/j.cgh.2013.09.023.

[15] Charlton, MR; Burns, JM; Pedersen, RA; Watt, KD; Heimbach, JK; Dierkhising, RA. Frequency and outcomes of liver transplantation for nonalcoholic steatohepatitis in the United States. *Gastroenterology.*, 2011, 141(4), 1249-1253. doi:10.1053/j.gastro.2011.06.061.

[16] Afzali, A; Berry, K; Ioannou, GN. Excellent posttransplant survival for patients with nonalcoholic steatohepatitis in the United States. *Liver Transplant.*, 2012, 18(1), 29-37. doi:10.1002/lt.22435.

[17] Cholankeril, G; Wong, RJ; Hu, M; et al. Liver Transplantation for Nonalcoholic Steatohepatitis in the US: Temporal Trends and Outcomes. *Dig Dis Sci.*, 2017, 62(10), 2915-2922. doi:10.1007/s10620-017-4684-x.

[18] Wong, RJ; Chou, C; Bonham, CA; Concepcion, W; Esquivel, CO; Ahmed, A. Improved survival outcomes in patients with non-alcoholic steatohepatitis and alcoholic liver disease following liver transplantation: an analysis of 2002-2012 United Network for Organ Sharing data. *Clin Transplant.*, 2014, 28(6), 713-721. doi:10.1111/ctr.12364.

[19] Singal, AK; Hasanin, M; Kaif, M; Wiesner, R; Kuo, YF. Nonalcoholic Steatohepatitis is the Most Rapidly Growing Indication for Simultaneous Liver Kidney Transplantation in the United States. *Transplantation.*, 2016, 100(3), 607-612. doi:10.1097/ TP.00000000 00000945.

[20] Kemmer, N; Neff, GW; Franco, E; et al. Nonalcoholic Fatty Liver Disease Epidemic and Its Implications for Liver Transplantation. *Transplantation.*, October 2013, 1. doi:10.1097/ 01.tp.0000436723. 59879.01.

[21] Agopian, VG; Kaldas, FM; Hong, JC; et al. Liver Transplantation for Nonalcoholic Steatohepatitis. *Ann Surg.*, 2012, 256(4), 624-633. doi:10.1097/SLA.0b013e31826b4b7e.

[22] Barritt, AS; Dellon, ES; Kozlowski, T; Gerber, DA; Hayashi, PH. The influence of nonalcoholic fatty liver disease and its associated comorbidities on liver transplant outcomes. *J Clin Gastroenterol.*, 2011, 45(4), 372-378. doi:10.1097/MCG.0b013e3181eeaff0.

[23] Wadden, TA; Volger, S; Sarwer, DB; et al. A two-year randomized trial of obesity treatment in primary care practice. *N Engl J Med.*, 2011, 365(21), 1969-1979. doi:10.1056/NEJMoa1109220.

[24] Romero-Gómez, M; Zelber-Sagi, S; Trenell, M. Treatment of NAFLD with diet, physical activity and exercise. *J Hepatol.*, 2017, 67(4), 829-846. doi:10.1016/j.jhep.2017.05.016.

[25] Rabl, C; Campos, GM. The impact of bariatric surgery on nonalcoholic steatohepatitis. *Semin Liver Dis.*, 2012, 32(1), 80-91. doi:10.1055/s-0032-1306428.

[26] Weiner, RA. Surgical Treatment of Non-Alcoholic Steatohepatitis and Non-Alcoholic Fatty Liver Disease. *Dig Dis.*, 2010, 28(1), 274-279. doi:10.1159/000282102.

[27] Furuya, CK; de Oliveira, CPMS; de Mello, ES; et al. Effects of bariatric surgery on nonalcoholic fatty liver disease: preliminary findings after 2 years. *J Gastroenterol Hepatol.*, 2007, 22(4), 510-514. doi:10.1111/j.1440-1746.2007.04833.x.

[28] Buchwald, H; Williams, SE. Bariatric surgery worldwide 2003. *Obes Surg.*, 2004, 14(9), 1157-1164. doi:10.1381/0960892042387057.

[29] Rogers, CC; Alloway, RR; Alexander, JW; Cardi, M; Trofe, J; Vinks, AA. Pharmacokinetics of mycophenolic acid, tacrolimus and sirolimus after gastric bypass surgery in end-stage renal disease and transplant patients: a pilot study. *Clin Transplant.*, 2007, 22(3), 281-291. doi:10.1111/j.1399-0012.2007.00783.x.

[30] Diwan, TS; Lichvar, AB; Leino, AD; et al. Pharmacokinetic and pharmacogenetic analysis of immunosuppressive agents after laparoscopic sleeve gastrectomy. *Clin Transplant.*, 2017, 31(6), e12975. doi:10.1111/ctr.12975.

[31] Clinical Guidelines on the Identification, Evaluation, and Treatment of Overweight and Obesity in Adults--The Evidence Report. National Institutes of Health. *Obes Res.*, 1998, 6 Suppl, 2, 51S-209S. http://www.ncbi.nlm.nih.gov/pubmed/9813653. Accessed June 9, 2019.

[32] Tsochatzis, E; Coilly, A; Nadalin, S; et al. International Liver Transplantation Consensus Statement on End-stage Liver Disease Due to Nonalcoholic Steatohepatitis and Liver Transplantation. *Transplantation.*, 2019, 103(1), 45-56. doi:10.1097/ TP.00000000 00002433.

[33] Sadler, EM; Mehta, N; Bhat, M; et al. Liver Transplantation for NASH-Related Hepatocellular Carcinoma Versus Non-NASH Etiologies of Hepatocellular Carcinoma. *Transplantation.*, 2018, 102(4), 640-647. doi:10.1097/TP.0000000000002043.

[34] Vanwagner, LB; Bhave, M; Te, HS; Feinglass, J; Alvarez, L; Rinella, ME. Patients transplanted for nonalcoholic steatohepatitis are at increased risk for postoperative cardiovascular events. *Hepatology.*, 2012, 56(5), 1741-1750. doi:10.1002/hep.25855.

[35] Bhagat, V; Mindikoglu, AL; Nudo, CG; Schiff, ER; Tzakis, A; Regev, A. Outcomes of liver transplantation in patients with cirrhosis

due to nonalcoholic steatohepatitis versus patients with cirrhosis due to alcoholic liver disease. *Liver Transpl.*, 2009, 15(12), 1814-1820. doi:10.1002/lt.21927.

[36] Kennedy, C; Redden, D; Gray, S; et al. Equivalent survival following liver transplantation in patients with non-alcoholic steatohepatitis compared with patients with other liver diseases. *HPB* (Oxford)., 2012, 14(9), 625-634. doi:10.1111/j.1477-2574.2012.00497.x.

[37] Malik, SM; deVera, ME; Fontes, P; Shaikh, O; Ahmad, J. Outcome after liver transplantation for NASH cirrhosis. *Am J Transplant.*, 2009, 9(4), 782-793. doi:10.1111/j.1600-6143.2009.02590.x.

[38] Bosch, J; Harrison, SA; Abdelmalek, MF et al. Hepatic Venous Pressure Gradient Predicts Clinical Disease Progression in Patients With Compensated Cirrhosis Due to Nonalcoholic Steatohepatitis. *Hepatology.*, 2017, 66, 244A. http://www.natap.org/2017/ AASLD/ AASLD_99.htm.

[39] Hui, JM; Kench, JG; Chitturi, S; et al. Long-term outcomes of cirrhosis in nonalcoholic steatohepatitis compared with hepatitis C. *Hepatology.*, 2003, 38(2), 420-427. doi:10.1053/jhep.2003.50320.

[40] Yatsuji, S; Hashimoto, E; Tobari, M; Taniai, M; Tokushige, K; Shiratori, K. Clinical features and outcomes of cirrhosis due to non-alcoholic steatohepatitis compared with cirrhosis caused by chronic hepatitis C. *J Gastroenterol Hepatol.*, 2009, 24(2), 248-254. doi:10.1111/j.1440-1746.2008.05640.x.

[41] Sanyal, AJ; Banas, C; Sargeant, C; et al. Similarities and differences in outcomes of cirrhosis due to nonalcoholic steatohepatitis and hepatitis C. *Hepatology.*, 2006, 43(4), 682-689. doi:10.1002/ hep.21103.

[42] O'Leary, JG; Landaverde, C; Jennings, L; Goldstein, RM; Davis, GL. Patients with NASH and cryptogenic cirrhosis are less likely than those with hepatitis C to receive liver transplants. *Clin Gastroenterol Hepatol.*, 2011, 9(8), 700-704.e1. doi:10.1016/ j.cgh.2011.04.007.

[43] Young, K; Aguilar, M; Gish, R; et al. Lower rates of receiving model for end-stage liver disease exception and longer time to transplant

among nonalcoholic steatohepatitis hepatocellular carcinoma. *Liver Transpl.*, 2016, 22(10), 1356-1366. doi:10.1002/lt.24507.

[44] Houlihan, DD; Armstrong, MJ; Davidov, Y; et al. Renal function in patients undergoing transplantation for nonalcoholic steatohepatitis cirrhosis: Time to reconsider immunosuppression regimens? *Liver Transplant.*, 2011, 17(11), 1292-1298. doi:10.1002/lt.22382.

[45] Park, CW; Tsai, NT; Wong, LL. Implications of worse renal dysfunction and medical comorbidities in patients with NASH undergoing liver transplant evaluation: impact on MELD and more. *Clin Transplant.*, 2011, 25(6), E606-11. doi:10.1111/j.1399-0012.2011.01497.x.

[46] Lonardo, A; Nascimbeni, F; Mantovani, A; Targher, G. Hypertension, diabetes, atherosclerosis and NASH: Cause or consequence? *J Hepatol.*, 2018, 68(2), 335-352. doi:10.1016/ j.jhep.2017.09.021.

[47] Targher, G; Byrne, CD; Lonardo, A; Zoppini, G; Barbui, C. Non-alcoholic fatty liver disease and risk of incident cardiovascular disease: A meta-analysis. *J Hepatol.*, 2016, 65(3), 589-600. doi:10.1016/ j.jhep.2016.05.013.

[48] Manoushagian, S; Meshkov, A. Evaluation of solid organ transplant candidates for coronary artery disease. *Am J Transplant.*, 2014, 14(10), 2228-2234. doi:10.1111/ajt.12915.

[49] Targher, G; Bertolini, L; Padovani, R; et al. Increased prevalence of cardiovascular disease in Type 2 diabetic patients with non-alcoholic fatty liver disease. *Diabet Med.*, 2006, 23(4), 403-409. doi:10.1111/j. 1464-5491.2006.01817.x.

[50] Arslan, U; Türkoğlu, S; Balcioğlu, S; Tavil, Y; Karakan, T; Cengel, A. Association between nonalcoholic fatty liver disease and coronary artery disease. *Coron Artery Dis.*, 2007, 18(6), 433-436. doi:10.1097/MCA.0b013e3282583c0d.

[51] Choi, SY; Kim, D; Kim, HJ; et al. The relation between non-alcoholic fatty liver disease and the risk of coronary heart disease in Koreans. *Am J Gastroenterol.*, 2009, 104(8), 1953-1960. doi:10.1038/ ajg.2009.238.

[52] Lu, H; Zeng, L; Liang, B; Shu, X; Xie, D. High prevalence of coronary heart disease in type 2 diabetic patients with non-alcoholic fatty liver disease. *Arch Med Res.*, 2009, 40(7), 571-575. doi:10.1016/j. arcmed.2009.07.009.

[53] Plotkin, JS; Johnson, LB; Rustgi, V; Kuo, PC. Coronary artery disease and liver transplantation: the state of the art. *Liver Transpl.*, 2000, 6(4 Suppl 1), S53-6. doi:[not.

[54] Chalasani, N; Younossi, Z; Lavine, JE; et al. The diagnosis and management of nonalcoholic fatty liver disease: Practice guidance from the American Association for the Study of Liver Diseases. *Hepatology.*, 2018, 67(1), 328-357. doi:10.1002/hep.29367.

[55] Vargas, JI; Arrese, M; Shah, VH; Arab, JP. Use of Statins in Patients with Chronic Liver Disease and Cirrhosis: Current Views and Prospects. *Curr Gastroenterol Rep.*, 2017, 19(9), 43. doi:10.1007/s11894-017-0584-7.

[56] Dongiovanni, P; Petta, S; Mannisto, V; et al. Statin use and non-alcoholic steatohepatitis in at risk individuals. *J Hepatol.*, 2015, 63(3), 705-712. doi:10.1016/j.jhep.2015.05.006.

[57] Fernández-Miranda, C; Pérez-Carreras, M; Colina, F; López-Alonso, G; Vargas, C; Solís-Herruzo, JA. A pilot trial of fenofibrate for the treatment of non-alcoholic fatty liver disease. *Dig Liver Dis.*, 2008, 40(3), 200-205. doi:10.1016/j.dld.2007.10.002.

[58] Goh, GB; Pagadala, MR; Dasarathy, J; et al. Renin-angiotensin system and fibrosis in non-alcoholic fatty liver disease. *Liver Int.*, 2015, 35(3), 979-985. doi:10.1111/liv.12611.

[59] Musso, G; Gambino, R; Tabibian, JH; et al. Association of non-alcoholic fatty liver disease with chronic kidney disease: a systematic review and meta-analysis. Woodward M, ed. *PLoS Med.*, 2014, 11(7), e1001680. doi:10.1371/journal.pmed.1001680.

[60] Di Maira, T; Rubin, A; Puchades, L; et al. Framingham score, renal dysfunction, and cardiovascular risk in liver transplant patients. *Liver Transpl.*, 2015, 21(6), 812-822. doi:10.1002/lt.24128.

[61] VanWagner, LB; Montag, S; Zhao, L; et al. Cardiovascular Disease Outcomes Related to Early Stage Renal Impairment After Liver

Transplantation. *Transplantation.*, 2018, 102(7), 1096-1107. doi:10.1097/TP.0000000000002175.

[62] VanWagner, LB; Ning, H; Whitsett, M; et al. A point-based prediction model for cardiovascular risk in orthotopic liver transplantation: The CAR-OLT score. *Hepatology.*, 2017, 66(6), 1968-1979. doi:10.1002/ hep.29329.

[63] Alvarez-Sotomayor, D; Satorres, C; Rodríguez-Medina, B; et al. Controlling Diabetes After Liver Transplantation: Room for Improvement. *Transplantation.*, 2016, 100(10), e66-e73. doi:10.1097/ TP.0000000000001399.

[64] Martínez-Saldivar, B; Prieto, J; Berenguer, M; et al. Control of blood pressure in liver transplant recipients. *Transplantation.*, 2012, 93(10), 1031-1037. doi:10.1097/TP.0b013e31824cd5e6.

[65] Dunkelgrun, M; Boersma, E; Schouten, O; et al. Bisoprolol and fluvastatin for the reduction of perioperative cardiac mortality and myocardial infarction in intermediate-risk patients undergoing noncardiovascular surgery: a randomized controlled trial (DECREASE-IV). *Ann Surg.*, 2009, 249(6), 921-926. doi:10.1097/ SLA.0b013e3181a77d00.

[66] Hindler, K; Shaw, AD; Samuels, J; Fulton, S; Collard, CD; Riedel, B. Improved postoperative outcomes associated with preoperative statin therapy. *Anesthesiology.*, 2006, 105(6), 1260-1272, quiz 1289-1290. http://www.ncbi.nlm.nih.gov/pubmed/17122590. Accessed June 9; 2019.

[67] Lewis, JH; Mortensen, ME; Zweig, S; et al. Efficacy and safety of high-dose pravastatin in hypercholesterolemic patients with well-compensated chronic liver disease: Results of a prospective, randomized, double-blind, placebo-controlled, multicenter trial. *Hepatology.*, 2007, 46(5), 1453-1463. doi:10.1002/hep.21848.

[68] Berzigotti, A; Saran, U; Dufour, JF. Physical activity and liver diseases. *Hepatology.*, 2016, 63(3), 1026-1040. doi:10.1002/ hep.28132.

[69] Berzigotti, A; Albillos, A; Villanueva, C; et al. Effects of an intensive lifestyle intervention program on portal hypertension in patients with

cirrhosis and obesity: The SportDiet study. *Hepatology.*, 2017, 65(4), 1293-1305. doi:10.1002/hep.28992.

[70] Leibovitz, E; Giryes, S; Makhline, R; Zikri Ditch, M; Berlovitz, Y; Boaz, M. Malnutrition risk in newly hospitalized overweight and obese individuals: Mr NOI. *Eur J Clin Nutr.*, 2013, 67(6), 620-624. doi:10.1038/ejcn.2013.45.

[71] Debette-Gratien, M; Tabouret, T; Antonini, MT; et al. Personalized adapted physical activity before liver transplantation: acceptability and results. *Transplantation.*, 2015, 99(1), 145-150. doi:10.1097/TP.0000000000000245.

[72] Zenith, L; Meena, N; Ramadi, A; et al. Eight weeks of exercise training increases aerobic capacity and muscle mass and reduces fatigue in patients with cirrhosis. *Clin Gastroenterol Hepatol.*, 2014, 12(11), 1920-6.e2. doi:10.1016/j.cgh.2014.04.016.

[73] Leonard, J; Heimbach, JK; Malinchoc, M; Watt, K; Charlton, M. The impact of obesity on long-term outcomes in liver transplant recipients-results of the NIDDK liver transplant database. *Am J Transplant.*, 2008, 8(3), 667-672. doi:10.1111/j.1600-6143.2007.02100.x.

[74] Wong, RJ; Cheung, R; Perumpail, RB; Holt, EW; Ahmed, A. Diabetes mellitus, and not obesity, is associated with lower survival following liver transplantation. *Dig Dis Sci.*, 2015, 60(4), 1036-1044. doi:10.1007/s10620-014-3469-8.

[75] Dick, AAS; Spitzer, AL; Seifert, CF; et al. Liver transplantation at the extremes of the body mass index. *Liver Transpl.*, 2009, 15(8), 968-977. doi:10.1002/lt.21785.

[76] Kardashian, AA; Dodge, JL; Roberts, J; Brandman, D. Weighing the risks: Morbid obesity and diabetes are associated with increased risk of death on the liver transplant waiting list. *Liver Int.*, 2018, 38(3), 553-563. doi:10.1111/liv.13523.

[77] Saab, S; Lalezari, D; Pruthi, P; Alper, T; Tong, MJ. The impact of obesity on patient survival in liver transplant recipients: a meta-analysis. *Liver Int.*, 2015, 35(1), 164-170. doi:10.1111/liv.12431.

[78] Barone, M; Viggiani, MT; Avolio, AW; Iannone, A; Rendina, M; Di Leo, A. Obesity as predictor of postoperative outcomes in liver transplant candidates: Review of the literature and future perspectives. *Dig Liver Dis.*, 2017, 49(9), 957-966. doi:10.1016/j.dld.2017.07.004.

[79] Rustgi, VK; Marino, G; Rustgi, S; et al. Impact of body mass index on graft failure and overall survival following liver transplant. *Clin Transplant.*, 2004, 18(6), 634-637. doi:10.1111/j.1399-0012.2004.00141.x.

[80] Conzen, KD; Vachharajani, N; Collins, KM; et al. Morbid obesity in liver transplant recipients adversely affects longterm graft and patient survival in a single-institution analysis. *HPB* (Oxford)., 2015, 17(3), 251-257. doi:10.1111/hpb.12340.

[81] Pelletier, SJ; Maraschio, MA; Schaubel, DE; et al. Survival benefit of kidney and liver transplantation for obese patients on the waiting list. *Clin Transpl.*, 2003, 77-88. http://www.ncbi.nlm.nih.gov/pubmed/15387099. Accessed June 9; 2019.

[82] Singhal, A; Wilson, GC; Wima, K; et al. Impact of recipient morbid obesity on outcomes after liver transplantation. *Transpl Int.*, 2015, 28(2), 148-155. doi:10.1111/tri.12483.

[83] Younossi, ZM; Stepanova, M; Saab, S; et al. The impact of type 2 diabetes and obesity on the long-term outcomes of more than 85 000 liver transplant recipients in the US. *Aliment Pharmacol Ther.*, 2014, 40(6), 686-694. doi:10.1111/apt.12881.

[84] Dare, AJ; Plank, LD; Phillips, ARJ; et al. Additive effect of pretransplant obesity, diabetes, and cardiovascular risk factors on outcomes after liver transplantation. *Liver Transpl.*, 2014, 20(3), 281-290. doi:10.1002/lt.23818.

[85] Sjöström, L; Lindroos, AK; Peltonen, M; et al. Lifestyle, diabetes, and cardiovascular risk factors 10 years after bariatric surgery. *N Engl J Med.*, 2004, 351(26), 2683-2693. doi:10.1056/ NEJMoa035622.

[86] Maggard, MA; Shugarman, LR; Suttorp, M; et al. Meta-analysis: surgical treatment of obesity. *Ann Intern Med.*, 2005, 142(7), 547-

559. http://www.ncbi.nlm.nih.gov/pubmed/15809466. Accessed June 9, 2019.

[87] McTigue, KM; Harris, R; Hemphill, B; et al. Screening and interventions for obesity in adults: summary of the evidence for the U.S. Preventive Services Task Force. *Ann Intern Med.*, 2003, 139(11), 933-949. http://www.ncbi.nlm.nih.gov/pubmed/14644897. Accessed June 9, 2019.

[88] Ma, Y; Pagoto, S; Olendzki, B; et al. Predictors of Weight Status following Laparoscopic Gastric Bypass. *Obes Surg.*, 2006, 16(9), 1227-1231. doi:10.1381/096089206778392284.

[89] Schauer, PR; Bhatt, DL; Kirwan, JP; et al. Bariatric Surgery versus Intensive Medical Therapy for Diabetes — 3-Year Outcomes. *N Engl J Med.*, 2014, 370(21), 2002-2013. doi:10.1056/NEJMoa1401329.

[90] Maciejewski, ML; Arterburn, DE; Van Scoyoc, L; et al. Bariatric Surgery and Long-term Durability of Weight Loss. *JAMA Surg.*, 2016, 151(11), 1046-1055. doi:10.1001/jamasurg.2016.2317.

[91] Murali, SB. Long-term Survival Following Bariatric Surgery in the VA Health System. *JAMA.*, 2015, 313(14), 1473. doi:10.1001/jama.2015.2580.

[92] Adams, TD; Stroup, AM; Gress, RE; et al. Cancer Incidence and Mortality After Gastric Bypass Surgery. *Obesity.*, 2009, 17(4), 796-802. doi:10.1038/oby.2008.610.

[93] Sjöström, L; Gummesson, A; Sjöström, CD; et al. Effects of bariatric surgery on cancer incidence in obese patients in Sweden (Swedish Obese Subjects Study): a prospective, controlled intervention trial. *Lancet Oncol.*, 2009, 10(7), 653-662. doi:10.1016/S1470-2045(09)70159-7.

[94] Young, MT; Gebhart, A; Phelan, MJ; Nguyen, NT. Use and Outcomes of Laparoscopic Sleeve Gastrectomy vs Laparoscopic Gastric Bypass: Analysis of the American College of Surgeons NSQIP. *J Am Coll Surg.*, 2015, 220(5), 880-885. doi:10.1016/j.jamcollsurg.2015.01.059.

[95] Himpens, J; Dapri, G; Cadière, GB. A prospective randomized study between laparoscopic gastric banding and laparoscopic isolated

sleeve gastrectomy: results after 1 and 3 years. *Obes Surg.*, 2006, 16(11), 1450-1456. doi:10.1381/096089206778869933.

[96] Nguyen, NT; Nguyen, B; Gebhart, A; Hohmann, S. Changes in the makeup of bariatric surgery: a national increase in use of laparoscopic sleeve gastrectomy. *J Am Coll Surg.*, 2013, 216(2), 252-257. doi:10.1016/j.jamcollsurg.2012.10.003.

[97] Lazzati, A; Iannelli, A; Schneck, AS; et al. Bariatric surgery and liver transplantation: a systematic review a new frontier for bariatric surgery. *Obes Surg.*, 2015, 25(1), 134-142. doi:10.1007/s11695-014-1430-8.

[98] Lazzati, A; Guy-Lachuer, R; Delaunay, V; Szwarcensztein, K; Azoulay, D. Bariatric surgery trends in France: 2005-2011. *Surg Obes Relat Dis.*, 2014, 10(2), 328-334. doi:10.1016/ j.soard.2013.07.015.

[99] Shimizu, H; Phuong, V; Maia, M; et al. Bariatric surgery in patients with liver cirrhosis. *Surg Obes Relat Dis.*, 2013, 9(1), 1-6. doi:10.1016/j.soard.2012.07.021.

[100] Dallal, RM; Mattar, SG; Lord, JL; et al. Results of Laparoscopic Gastric Bypass in Patients with Cirrhosis. *Obes Surg.*, 2004, 14(1), 47-53. doi:10.1381/096089204772787284.

[101] Tariq, N; Moore, LW; Sherman, V. Bariatric Surgery and End-Stage Organ Failure. *Surg Clin North Am.*, 2013, 93(6), 1359-1371. doi:10.1016/j.suc.2013.08.006.

[102] Takata, MC; Campos, GM; Ciovica, R; et al. Laparoscopic bariatric surgery improves candidacy in morbidly obese patients awaiting transplantation. *Surg Obes Relat Dis.*, 2008, 4(2), 159-164, discussion 164-5. doi:10.1016/j.soard.2007.12.009.

[103] Zamora-Valdes, D; Watt, KD; Kellogg, TA; et al. Long-term outcomes of patients undergoing simultaneous liver transplantation and sleeve gastrectomy. *Hepatology.*, 2018, 68(2), 485-495. doi:10.1002/hep.29848.

[104] Carson, K; Washington, MK; Treem, WR; Clavien, PA; Hunt, CM. Recurrence of nonalcoholic steatohepatitis in a liver transplant recipient. *Liver Transpl Surg.*, 1997, 3(2), 174-176. http://www.ncbi.nlm.nih.gov/pubmed/9346732. Accessed June 9; 2019.

[105] Lin, MYC; Tavakol, MM; Sarin, A; et al. Laparoscopic sleeve gastrectomy is safe and efficacious for pretransplant candidates. *Surg Obes Relat Dis.*, 2013, 9(5), 653-658. doi:10.1016/ j.soard. 2013.02.013.

[106] Braunfeld, MY; Chan, S; Pregler, J; et al. Liver transplantation in the morbidly obese. *J Clin Anesth.*, 1996, 8(7), 585-590. http:// www.ncbi.nlm.nih.gov/pubmed/8910182. Accessed June 9, 2019.

[107] Heimbach, JK; Watt, KDS; Poterucha, JJ; et al. Combined liver transplantation and gastric sleeve resection for patients with medically complicated obesity and end-stage liver disease. *Am J Transplant.*, 2013, 13(2), 363-368. doi:10.1111/j.1600-6143.2012.04318.x.

[108] Tariciotti, L; D'Ugo, S; Manzia, TM; et al. Combined liver transplantation and sleeve gastrectomy for end-stage liver disease in a bariatric patient: First European case-report. *Int J Surg Case Rep.*, 2016, 28, 38-41. doi:10.1016/j.ijscr.2016.09.011.

[109] Nesher, E; Mor, E; Shlomai, A; et al. Simultaneous Liver Transplantation and Sleeve Gastrectomy: Prohibitive Combination or a Necessity? *Obes Surg.*, 2017, 27(5), 1387-1390. doi:10.1007/ s11695-017-2634-5.

[110] Schlansky, B; Naugler, WE; Orloff, SL; Enestvedt, CK. Higher Mortality and Survival Benefit in Obese Patients Awaiting Liver Transplantation. *Transplantation.*, 2016, 100(12), 2648-2655. doi:10.1097/TP.0000000000001461.

[111] Bambha, KM; Dodge, JL; Gralla, J; Sprague, D; Biggins, SW. Low, rather than high, body mass index confers increased risk for post-liver transplant death and graft loss: Risk modulated by model for end-stage liver disease. *Liver Transplant.*, 2015, 21(10), 1286-1294. doi:10.1002/lt.24188.

[112] Perez-Protto, SE; Quintini, C; Reynolds, LF; et al. Comparable graft and patient survival in lean and obese liver transplant recipients. *Liver Transplant.*, 2013, 19(8), 907-915. doi:10.1002/lt.23680.

[113] Orci, LA; Majno, PE; Berney, T; Morel, P; Mentha, G; Toso, C. The impact of wait list body mass index changes on the outcome after liver

transplantation. *Transpl Int.*, 2013, 26(2), 170-176. doi:10.1111/ tri.12017.

[114] Watt, KDS; Charlton, MR. Metabolic syndrome and liver transplantation: a review and guide to management. *J Hepatol.*, 2010, 53(1), 199-206. doi:10.1016/j.jhep.2010.01.040.

[115] Nolan, JJ; Færch, K. Estimating insulin sensitivity and beta cell function: perspectives from the modern pandemics of obesity and type 2 diabetes. *Diabetologia.*, 2012, 55(11), 2863-2867. doi:10.1007/ s00125-012-2684-0.

[116] Executive Summary: Standards of Medical Care in Diabetes--2014. *Diabetes Care.*, 2014, 37(Supplement_1), S5-S13. doi:10.2337/dc14-S005.

[117] Tsamalaidze, L; Stauffer, JA; Arasi, LC; et al. Laparoscopic Sleeve Gastrectomy for Morbid Obesity in Patients After Orthotopic Liver Transplant: a Matched Case-Control Study. *Obes Surg.*, 2018, 28(2), 444-450. doi:10.1007/s11695-017-2847-7.

[118] Tichansky, DS; Madan, AK. Laparoscopic Roux-en-Y gastric bypass is safe and feasible after orthotopic liver transplantation. *Obes Surg.*, 2005, 15(10), 1481-1486. doi:10.1381/ 096089205774859164.

[119] Osseis, M; Lazzati, A; Salloum, C; et al. Sleeve Gastrectomy After Liver Transplantation: Feasibility and Outcomes. *Obes Surg.*, 2018, 28(1), 242-248. doi:10.1007/s11695-017-2843-y.

[120] Butte, JM; Devaud, N; Jarufe, NP; et al. Sleeve gastrectomy as treatment for severe obesity after orthotopic liver transplantation. *Obes Surg.*, 2007, 17(11), 1517-1519. http://www.ncbi.nlm.nih.gov/ pubmed/18219781. Accessed June 9, 2019.

[121] Elli, EF; Masrur, MA; Giulianotti, PC. Robotic sleeve gastrectomy after liver transplantation. *Surg Obes Relat Dis.*, 2013, 9(1), e20-e22. doi:10.1016/j.soard.2012.01.010.

[122] Wong, RJ; Aguilar, M; Cheung, R; et al. Nonalcoholic steatohepatitis is the second leading etiology of liver disease among adults awaiting liver transplantation in the United States. *Gastroenterology.*, 2015, 148(3), 547-555. doi:10.1053/j.gastro.2014.11.039.

[123] Yalamanchili, K; Saadeh, S; Klintmalm, GB; Jennings, LW; Davis, GL. Nonalcoholic fatty liver disease after liver transplantation for cryptogenic cirrhosis or nonalcoholic fatty liver disease. *Liver Transpl.*, 2010, 16(4), 431-439. doi:10.1002/lt.22004.

[124] Hakeem, AR; Cockbain, AJ; Raza, SS; et al. Increased morbidity in overweight and obese liver transplant recipients: a single-center experience of 1325 patients from the United Kingdom. *Liver Transpl.*, 2013, 19(5), 551-562. doi:10.1002/lt.23618.

[125] LaMattina, JC; Foley, DP; Fernandez, LA; et al. Complications associated with liver transplantation in the obese recipient. *Clin Transplant.*, 2012, 26(6), 910-918. doi:10.1111/j.1399-0012.2012.01669.x.

In: Liver Steatosis and Bariatric Surgery ISBN: 978-1-53616-444-2
Editors: Jaime Ruiz-Tovar et al.

Chapter 14

NON-SURGICAL TREATMENT OF NASH: THE OTHER OPTIONS

Raúl Bernal-Reyes[1,*], MD
and Daniel Bernal-Serrano[2], MD
[1]School of Medicine UNAM, Mexico City, Mexico
Gastroenterologist from National Medical Center IMSS,
Mexico City, Mexico
Gastroenterology Consultant at the Spanish Charitable Society,
Pachuca, Mexico
[2]International Adjunct Professor, Medical School,
Instituto Tecnológico y de Ciencias Superiores de Monterrey,
Mexico City, Mexico
MSc Health Policy, Planning and Financing candidate,
London School of Hygiene and Tropical Medicine & London School of
Economics and Political Science, London, UK.
Internal Medicine Specialist, Posgraduate Unit,
Universidad Nacional Autónoma de México, Mexico City, Mexico

[*] Corresponding Author's Email: raulber@yahoo.com.

ABSTRACT

The best result so far in the non-surgical treatment of NASH has been obtained with diet and physical activity supervised by professionals, this promotes the reduction of body weight and metabolic stabilization. The use of pharmacotherapy is only for patients with NASH in very specific contexts. For example, Pioglitazone and vitamin E can be used, since they have shown acceptable results according to various guides and consensus. Novel medications have shown encouraging results with positive effects in basic science studies or small clinical trials; studies with a larger number of patients and a more rigorous methodology are needed.

Keywords: medical-treatment of NASH, diet, exercise, clinical trials, experimental drugs, pioglitazone, vitamin E

INTRODUCTION

The prevalence of Non-Alcoholic Fatty Liver Disease (NAFLD) has peaked in the last 30 years. This worldwide epidemic has drawn the attention of diverse research groups that, by delving into the pathophysiology of the disease, have revealed the complex details of the disease. In its original description, the histopathological resemblance to alcoholic steato-hepatitis was highlighted [1]; however, the patients with NAFLD have low alcohol consumption: less than 30 grams per day in men, and less than 20 grams per day in women [2]. Ever since Ludwing's article was published in 1980, knowledge about NAFLD has increased. Its physiopathology has been related to diverse factors: high-fat and high-carbohydrate diet, extreme sedentarism, intestinal dysbiosis, insulin resistance, and the activation of macrophages and pro-inflammatory agents, to name the most researched ones.

The notable increase in knowledge about this disease allows us to delve into the physio-pathological steps that represent multiple opportunities for therapeutic action. This recent research interest is one of the reasons why the amount of therapeutic options nowadays is so large. However, many of these options come from preliminary case reports, mostly anecdotal, with poor methodology and rarely reproducible.

This disease's complexity and its multiple comorbidities compel us to consider the treatment of NAFLD in a broader context, since this is not just a liver disease. In fact it is a systemic one, and it is one of the components of the Metabolic Syndrome (MetS). It is estimated that up to 90% of patients with NAFLD have at least one associated component of MetS, usually obesity, followed in frequency by diabetes mellitus type 2 (DM2), dyslipidemia and arterial hypertension. It is recognized that as a patient gathers more components of the MetS, her risk of suffering NAFLD is greater [3]. This explains why commonly these patients require multiple treatments aimed not only at preventing the progression of liver disease, but also at promoting metabolic stability and at limiting the risk of cardiovascular disease, the main cause of death among patients with NASH. Each patient with NAFLD has a clinical profile of its own that makes him different from others, and therefore requires an individualized treatment; what today is known as patient-centered medicine. This is a compelling reason that explains why, today, the possibility of a standardized treatment for patients with NAFLD is remote, and it is an incentive to research into personalized medicine alternatives.

Another factor to have in mind, for therapeutic purposes, is the natural evolution of the disease. Most patients affected by NAFLD have a good prognosis if they remain in the steatosis stage, or Non-Alcoholic Fatty Liver (NAFL). Luckily, these are the majority and an effective change in lifestyle (weigh reduction diet and physical exercise) will suffice to accomplish metabolic stabilization, and even reverse steatosis.

The phenotype of the patients with NASH is different from patients with NAFL stage. These patients have a greater tendency to progression; particularly those in whom fibrosis has started have the worst prognosis for the having liver cirrhosis [4]. Therefore, the efforts to find a useful drug have focused mainly on the control and regression of NASH's characteristic inflammation and fibrosis.

Save for a few exceptions, drug therapy is advised only in patients with biopsy supported NASH diagnosis [5].

The most relevant controlled clinical drug trials have a success rate of less than 50%; therefore, major regulatory agencies have not approved any pharmacological treatment for NASH. Only vitamin E and pioglitazone have shown a limited beneficial effect in very specific contexts; nevertheless, they have the disadvantage of relevant side effects. There is another group of drugs whose reports initially showed good results; however, these were not confirmed when more stringent trials were undertaken. Finally, there is a very promising third group of drugs that are currently in phase II and phase III studies, they act in different points of the complex pathophysiology of NASH and a lot is expected from them in the years to come.

So far, the best results in the treatment of patients affected with NAFLD have been achieved with significant lifestyle changes. A weight reduction diet combined with physical activity can reduce steatosis, inflammation, and even liver fibrosis. Additionally, lifestyle changes favours metabolic control and stabilization of the comorbidities that frequently accompany NAFLD.

WEIGHT LOSS

Although most patients with NAFLD are overweight or obese, there are also cases of non-obese patients, this variety is known as "*lean NAFLD*". In these patients the presence of other components of MetS is common [6]. This is the reason most of them benefit from weigh reduction, which favours metabolic control and limits hepatic steatosis [7].

The effectiveness of weight reduction has been demonstrated in patients with NAFLD and corroborated with liver biopsies before and after the intervention. A loss of 7% initial body weight achieved a reduction of ≥ 2 points in the NAFLD Activity Score (NAS), with an improvement of fibrosis of up to 50%. When the weight reduction reached ≥ 10%, the improvement or resolution of fibrosis went up to 80% [8]. In general terms, a weight reduction ≥ 3% is enough to significantly reduce steatosis; a weight loss ≥ 7% has an impact on the development of NASH, decreasing the inflammation and hepatocyte ballooning, and a loss ≥ 10% can reduce fibrosis.

Due to the current absence of an approved pharmacological treatment for patients with NASH the fundamental pillars of therapy are lifestyle changes, based on a personalized diet and supervised physical activation. Jointly these promote not only weight reduction, but also metabolic stability and, therefore, a significant reduction in steatosis, inflammation, and hepatic fibrosis. Despite good results, this change in habits is seldom long lasting, and difficulties to treatment attachment remain a problem in the management of these patients.

DIET

The so-called western diet has gradually become omnipresent around the world, replacing traditional diets. This diet is based on the consumption of large portions of fast food; an excess of saturated fats and refined sugars characterizes it. Of the later fructose stands out, which one is used indiscriminately in the food industry and causes hepatocellular damage through different routes [9].

A first goal of a weight loss diet should be to reduce caloric intake. Initially patients with overweight and obesity should be advised to reduced saturated fat and refined sugars, the recommended ratio of nutrients is of approximately 20% protein, 30% fat (predominantly monounsaturated), and 50% carbohydrates. The average fiber intake should be of 25-35 gr. per day. It is very important to let the patients know that they should avoid eating processed foods, particularly sweet drinks because of their high fructose content [10, 11].

The best example of a diet with good results is the Mediterranean diet. It comprises an abundant consumption of fish and poultry as proteins sources, lots of vegetables and fruits, moderate portions of cheese and cereals, olive oil and moderate wine consumption; additionally it implies a significant restriction of red meat, snacks and desserts [12, 13]. The main features of the Mediterranean diet are high-fiber and antioxidant content, as well as properly balanced portions lipid and unrefined sugars. Additionally, the diversity of suggested foods favours greater acceptance and adherence, unlike the irregular compliance that characterizes hypocaloric diets [14].

Ketogenic diet also has been proposed as treatment for NAFLD. It became popular several years ago in morbidly obese patients who were to undertake bariatric surgery, because of its rapid effect of weight loss. It is based on carbohydrate restriction to induce a higher consumption of body fat deposits as main energy source. In other words, it shifts metabolism from a glycolytic state to a lipolytic one as a consequence of carbohydrate shortage, and it uptakes fat as the main source of energy. However, even though this diet has been shown to contribute to body weight loss, it has been questioned for inconveniences such as favouring constipation and a poor attachment of patients due to multiple food restrictions. Recently two relevant facts emerged; the first, that promoting a rapid weight loss could favours an increase in hepatic steatosis, and, the second, that this diet requires vitamin and mineral supplementation [15].

Due to the frequent comorbidities that condition diverse clinical profiles in patients with NAFLD and the metabolic complexity represented by the dietary adjustment, The Mexican Consensus on NAFLD recommends dietary management of these patients to be customized and implemented by a nutritionist, who most consider among other things, the average energy expenditure of each patient [5].

EXERCISE

Physical activity favours the consumption of calories, and a properly executed exercise routine offers benefits in metabolic control and induces weight loss through the mobilization of fat deposits. Biochemical effects of exercise are many fold, among the most notable are reducing insulin resistance, improving lipid metabolism, endothelial function, blood glucose levels, and reducing pro-inflammatory activity, all are common alterations in the patient with NAFLD [16].

A recent systematic review revealed that exercise by itself, even without significant weight loss, can reduce hepatic steatosis in 20% to 30%, regardless of whether being aerobic or resistance exercise [17]. Notwithstanding this, exercise as the sole therapeutic measure is not enough and should be complemented with a proper diet to promote weight loss, the most effective intervention so far [18]. In adults the WHO recommends a moderate aerobic exercise routine of between 150 and 200 minutes per week [19]. As is the case for diet, a professional who advises the patient on the intensity and type of exercise to be performed by each patient should supervise this routine.

PHARMACOTHERAPY

Pharmacological treatment is not for all patients with NAFLD, it is crucial to establish that it is only indicated in patients with NASH and evidence of fibrosis ($F \geq 2$), or in those with a higher risk of progression (DM2, MetS, or persistently elevated ALT) [5]. The ideal treatment should address not only liver damage, but also the associated metabolic alterations: DM2, obesity and dyslipidaemia. Additionally, it should consider cardiovascular risk, since these comorbidities confer an increased risk of disease progression and premature death. Regarding the liver, the ideal drug should reduce hepatic inflammation, hepatocellular damage, correct insulin resistance, and have anti-fibrotic effects [20, 21].

As stated above, to date there is not a single effective and safe pharmacological treatment for all patients with NASH. Therefore, the proposed options are many folds, with very different mechanisms of action and contrasting results.

For the objectives of this review, we will divide the most relevant drugs into three groups:

A. Drugs with some favourable effect.
B. Drugs that are discouraged.
C. Promising drugs in pharmaceutical development

1. Drugs with Some Favourable Effect

Fundamentally two medications, pioglitazone and vitamin E, may be indicated in very specific contexts. The maximum level of histological improvement they have is close to 50%. Both have been evaluated in several studies; the PIVENS study stands out for its good methodology, it included patients with NASH without cirrhosis or diabetes, and obtained acceptable results [22].

Pioglitazone

This drug belongs to the thiazolidinedione family of drugs and is a treatment for DM2. It acts as a *PPAR*-γ receptor agonist with very interesting and diverse pharmacological effects: improvement of insulin sensitivity in adipose tissue, favours the deposit of free fatty acids in adipose tissue instead of in the liver, increases the production of adiponectin, and favours beta-oxidation of fatty acids in the hepatocyte; additionally it might have anti-inflammatory and anti-fibrotic effects [23].

Several adequately controlled trials, with follow-up periods of up to 18 months support its indication in some patients with NASH with or without DM2. They have reported improvement in insulin resistance and aminotransferase levels. Histologically, a significant decrease in steatosis, inflammation and ballooning injury has been shown in hepatocytes. Also, there is an improvement of fibrosis in variable ranges, with a 73% NAS improvement in treated patients vs 24% in those who received placebo; resolution of NASH has been reported in 47% to 51% of treated patients [22, 24-26].

It is important to note that thiazolidinediones also decrease in cardiovascular mortality and cerebrovascular events [27, 28].

This drug is usually well tolerated, although the reported side effects should be considered and discussed with patients. The most common of these is an increase in body weight [22, 26]; others are a putative, and controverted, such as an increased risk for bladder cancer [29, 30] and hip fracture in postmenopausal women due to decreased bone density [31].

Vitamin E

Because of its antioxidant effect, vitamin E has been proposed as an effective option for patients with NASH. Some studies have shown a reduction in steatosis and inflammation, even a reduction in hepatocyte ballooning degeneration [22] the latter was seen in a study of children [32]. However, no effect on fibrosis or resolution of NASH has been reported. Initially it was not recommended for patients with diabetes, however later studies confirmed its utility in them [33].

Like in the case of pioglitazone, this drug also has relevant side effects. The most important is an association between high doses of vitamin E (> 400 UI per day) and mortality [34]. Others adverse effects are an increased risk of prostate cancer and haemorrhagic stroke [35].

Other drugs have early positive results at the laboratory level or in small patient groups. Nevertheless, we lack good quality controlled clinical trials that supports its prescription in patients with NASH. However, some of them could be used to treat some of the frequent comorbidities; this is the case of liraglutide [36-37] and pentoxifylline [38]; this group complements with others like silymarin, silybin-phospatidylcholine, pirfenidone, ademetionine and probiotics. We expect controlled clinical trials to be carried out in the coming years to confirm their effectiveness or to disqualify their use. For now the evidence is insufficient and does not support the prescription to treat patients with NASH [5].

2. Drugs that are Discouraged

In this group are those drugs that initially had good expectations, but whose effectiveness was rejected in subsequent studies, therefore they are not indicated in the treatment of NASH. Among the best known are metformin [39], ursodeoxycholic acid [40, 41], omega-3 fatty acids [42], and fibrates [43, 44].

As previously mentioned, these drugs were launched with quite optimistic reports regarding their therapeutic utility; however, in these cases there is enough clinical evidence from clinical trials and meta-analysis that reject their benefit, or that failed to reproduce the initial results. Therefore, they are not relevant for treating NASH.

Some of these drugs can be used in patients with NAFLD for the management of other comorbidities, such as DM2 or dyslipidemia, but not for fatty liver.

3. Drugs in Development

There is a growing interest of the pharmaceutical industry in developing new medicines with good and definitive results in the treatment of NASH. Currently there are many molecules in development, some of them in stages as advanced as phase II and phase III, with surprising initial results. They are especially effective in stopping and reversing inflammation and fibrosis. The following is a selection based on their potential benefit and stage of development.

Obeticholic Acid

This is a semisynthetic derivate of chenodeoxycholic acid that works as agonist of farnesoid X receptor (FXR). It reduces the synthesis of bile acids in the liver, as well as lipogenesis and gluconeogenesis, and it stimulates beta-oxidation. In the FLINT study [45], compared obeticholic acid with placebo for 72 weeks; patients in the intervention arm had significant improvement in steatosis, inflammation, hepatocyte ballooning degeneration and fibrosis; a reduction in NAS ≥ 2 was obtained; higher than that observed in those who received placebo (45% vs. 21% RR 1.9 was achieved; 95% CI 1.3 - 2.8, $p < 0.0002$). A phase III study is currently underway to evaluate its impact on fibrosis. In the same way, similar analogues are in development. The main side effect that has been reported with this drug is pruritus, in up to 23% of those who received it, increased LDL and decreased HDL also have been observed.

Cenicriviroc

It is an antiretroviral that inhibits receptors 2 and 5 of chemokine CC, its use in HIV patients is also investigated; in preliminary studies it has shown good anti-inflammatory and anti-fibrotic effects. In the CENTAUR study [46], an interesting design with a two-year follow-up was implemented. The final results did not reveal significant changes in steatosis or ballooning injury; however, it is noteworthy to say that there was an improvement in fibrosis without NASH worsening and this one was well tolerated.

Elafibranor

It is a *PPAR-αδ* agonist with anti-inflammatory effect. Metabolically its main characteristic is to improve insulin sensitivity and glucose levels as well as to stabilize lipid metabolism. The GOLDEN-505 study showed a better effect in patients with basal NAS ≥ 4 and receiving a higher dose (120mg). In these patients improvement in aminotransferases, serum lipids, glucose and inflammatory markers with significant decrease in fibrosis stage were shown. Elafibranor was well tolerated, improved patient's cardiometabolic risk profile, but induced renal failure in seven patients [47].

Selonsertib

Preliminary reports in a murine model indicate that this inhibitor of the regulatory kinase of signal of apoptosis (ASK1) that promotes liver fibrosis has a good anti-fibrotic effect. This effect was confirmed in a controlled clinical trial that showed the best results among those who received a dose of 18 mg for 24 weeks, resulting in a reduction of ≥ 1 in the stage of fibrosis in 43% of the patients, and in 30% of those who received a lower dose (6mg) [48]. It was also studied in combination with GS-0976 an Acetyl-coA carboxylase (ACC) inhibitor to block the synthesis of fatty acids and reduce steatosis, with good results confirmed by Magnetic Resonance proton density fat fraction (MRI-PDFF) [49]. The phase III trial STELLAR 3 and 4 currently investigates its safety and effectiveness [50].

Emricasan

This drug inhibits caspase and has an anti-apoptotic effect. Preliminary reports found encouraging results with good anti-fibrotic effect in murine models. Currently phase II studies are running in patients with NASH and fibrosis [51].

Aramchol

This drug is a combination of arachidonic and cholic acids, it reduces the synthesis of fatty acids and triglyceride deposits and promotes the intracellular elimination of cholesterol. In a 3-month follow-up study Magnetic Resonance Spectroscopy confirmed that it effectively reduced hepatic steatosis. The drug was well tolerated and no significant side effects were reported [52], a phase IIb study is currently underway [53]. Aramchol has been granted a Fast Track designation status by the FDA for the treatment of NASH.

Combined Treatments

The inherent complexity of the NAFLD's pathophysiology suggests that it is unlikely that a single drug will achieve the best result. Hence, the individualization of treatment through the combination of drugs that allow us to intervene at different metabolic levels is required to stop the progression of the disease and reverse the present damage.

Currently there are few reports of this mixed therapy. An example is the combination of Selonsertib with Sintuzumab, reported by Loomba in a small group of patients; it showed that Sintuzumab achieved an improvement of ≥ 1 in fibrosis stage when combined with Selonsertib (6mg) in up to 40% of patients, compared with only 13% of those who were allocated to Sintuzumab alone [54].

There are other reports for the combination of vitamin E and vitamin C, in theory this dual therapy has the potential to reduce hepatic fibrosis [55]. Also, the combination of sitagliptin and losartan in a murine model was able to inhibit progression of disease [56].

These reports are preliminary and the currently available results for these combinations lack enough evidence to support its clinical use.

Controlled design studies with high quality scientific evidence in larger groups of patients are necessary to have solid clinical claims.

CONCLUSION

The alarming increase in the worldwide number of patients with NAFLD demands drugs that offer useful healing alternatives. However, since this is primarily a metabolic disease (associated with other components of the MetS) the variability of its clinical phenotypes is widespread and this limits the use of a universal drug in all patients. On the other hand, the better knowledge of the multiple and complex pathophysiology of this disease has allowed to develop multiple therapeutic proposals with encouraging results. However, until now, none of them has been approved by the main regulatory agencies.

The best result so far has been obtained with diet and physical activity supervised by professionals, this promotes the reduction of body weight and metabolic stabilization. Both interventions are recommended in patients with NAFL and with NASH.

The use of pharmacotherapy is only for patients with NASH in very specific contexts. Pioglitazone and vitamin E can be used, since they have shown acceptable results according to various guides and consensus. Other medications that have been proposed in preliminary studies, did not confirm their apparent benefits when subjected to more rigorous research methods. Therefore, today they are not recommended for the treatment of NASH; this is the case of metformin, omega-3 fatty acids and ursodeoxycholic acid.

Other novel medications have shown encouraging results with positive effects in basic science studies or small clinical trials; studies with a larger number of patients and a more rigorous methodology are expected to confirm their usefulness. Pirfenidone, liraglutide, silymarin, and probiotics are the most relevant of this group.

Finally, there is a very interesting group of drugs currently undertaking formal studies, with optimistic their initial results. The most relevant are obeticolic acid, cenicriviroc, elafibranor, selonsertib and aramchol. Almost all of them are in phase II and III studies, whose final reports are expected in the coming months.

Given the complexity of this disease, and the diverse clinical scenarios that each patient represents, combined treatment of two, or more drugs is emerging as the most viable therapeutic strategy. For now, in general terms, we hold that diet and exercise have proved useful in most cases and that the future with drug therapy is optimistic. Most likely we will have to combine them depending on each patient comorbidities. That is, we will have to make a suit tailored to each of our patients to achieve metabolic control, stop the progression of the disease, and reverse established liver damage as much as possible.

REFERENCES

[1] Ludwig, J; Viggiano, TR; McGill, DB; Ott, BJ. Nonalcoholic steatohepatitis, Mayo Clinc experience with a hitherto unnamed disease. *Mayo Clin Proc*, 1980, 55, 434-8.

[2] Ratziu, V; Bellentani, S; Cortez-Pinto, H; et al. A position statement on NAFLD/NASH based on the EASL 2009 special conference. *J Hepatol*, 2010, 53, 372-84.

[3] Ong, JP; Younossi, ZM. Epidemiology and Natural History of NAFLD and NASH. *Clin Liv Dis*, 2007, 11, 1-16.

[4] Angulo, P; Kleiner, DE; dam Larsen, S; et al. Liver fibrosis, but no other histologic features, is associated with long-term outcomes of patients with nonalcoholic fatty liver disease. *Gastroenterology*, 2015, 149(2), 389-97.

[5] Bernal-Reyes, R; Castro-Narro, G; Malé-Velázquez, R; et al. The Mexican Consensus on Nonalcoholic Fatty Liver Disease. *Rev Gastroenterol Mex*, 2019, 84(1), 69-99.

[6] Younes, R; Bugianesi, E. NASH in Lean Individuals. *Semin Liver Dis*, 2019, 39, 8695.

[7] Ohkawara, K; Tanaka, S; Miyachi, M; et al. A dose-response relation between aerobic exercise and visceral fat reduction: systematic review of clinical trials. *Int J Obes*, 2007, 31(12), 1786-1797.

[8] Vilar-Gomez, E; Martinez-Perez, Y; Calzadilla-Bertot, L; et al. Weight loss through lifestyle modification significantly reduces features of non-alcoholic steatohepatitis. *Gastroenterology*, 2015, 149, 367-78.

[9] Vos, MB; McClain, CJ. Fructose takes a toll. *Hepatology*, 2009, 50(4), 1004-06

[10] Brea, A; Pintó, X; Ascaso, JF; et al. Non-alcoholic fatty liver disease, association with cardiovascular disease and treatment (II). *Clin Investig Arterioscler*, 2017, 29, 185-200.

[11] Chalasani, N; Younossi, Z; Lavine, JE; et al. The diagnosis and management of non-alcoholic fatty liver disease: Practice guideline by the American Association for the Study of Liver Diseases, American College of Gastroenterology, and the American Gastroenterological Association. *Am J Gastroenterol*, 2012, 107, 811-26.

[12] Grosso, G; Mistretta, A; Frigiola, A; et al. Mediterranean diet and cardiovascular risk factors: a systematic review. *Crit Rev Food Sci Nutr*, 2014, 54, 593-610.

[13] European Association for the Study of the Liver (EASL), European Association for the Study of Diabetes (EASD), European Association for the Study of Obesity (EASO), EASL-EASD-EASO Clinical Practice Guidelines for the management of non-alcoholic fatty liver disease. *J Hepatol*, 2016, 64, 1388-402.

[14] Yki, Järvinen H. Nutritional modulation of non-alcoholic fatty liver disease and insulin resistance. *Nutrients*, 2015, 7(11), 9127-38.

[15] Gupta, L; Khandelwal, D; Kalra, S; et al. Ketogenic diet in endocrine disorders: Current Perspectives. *J Postgrad Med*, 2017, 63(4), 242-51.

[16] Romero-Gómez, M; Zelber-Sagi, S; Trenell, M. Treatment of NAFLD with diet, physical activity and exercise. *J Hepatol*, 2017, 67, 829-46.

[17] Hashida, R; Kawaguchi, T; Bekki, M; et al. Aerobic vs resistance exercise in non-alcoholic fatty liver disease: A systematic review. *J Hepatol*, 2017, 66, 142-152.

[18] Ueno, T; Sugawara, H; Sujaku, K; et al. Therapeutic effects of restricted diet and exercise in obese patients with fatty liver. *J Hepatol*, 1997, 27, 103-107.
[19] World Health Organization. Global Recommendations on physical ac tivity for health. *Geneva World Health Organization*, 2010.
[20] Mazzella, N; Ricciardi, LM; Mazzotti, A; et al. The role of medications for the management of patients with NAFLD. *Clin Liver Dis.*, 2014, 18, 73-89,
[21] Ratziu, V; Goodman, Z; Sanyal, A. Current efforts and trends in the treatment of NASH. *J Hepatol*, 2015, 62, S65-75.
[22] Sanyal, AJ; Chalasani, N; Kowdley, KV; et al. Pioglitazone, vitamin E, or placebo for nonalcoholic steatohepatitis. *N Engl J Med.*, 2010, 362, 1675-85.
[23] Liss, KH; Flinck, BN. PPARs and non-alcoholic fatty liver disease. *Biochimie*, 2017, 136, 65-74.
[24] Aithal, GP; Thomas, JA; Kaye, PV; et al. Randomized, placebo-controlled trial of pioglitazone in nondiabetic subjects with nonalcoholic steatohepatitis. *Gastroenterology*, 2008, 135, 1176-84.
[25] Belfort, R; Harrison, SA; Brown, K; et al. A placebo controlled trial of pioglitazone in subjects with nonalcoholic steatohepatitis. *N Engl J Med.*, 2006, 355, 2297-307.
[26] Cusi, K; Orsak, B; Bril, F; et al. Long-term pioglitazone treatment for patients with non-alcoholic steatohepatitis and prediabetes or type 2 diabetes mellitus: A randomized trial. *Ann Intern Med*, 2016, 165, 305-15.
[27] Lincoff, AM; Wolski, K; Nicholls, SJ; Nissen, SE. Pioglitazone and risk of cardiovascular events in patients with type 2 diabetes mellitus: a meta-analysis of randomized trials. *JAMA*, 2007, 298, 1180-8.
[28] Kernan, WN; Viscoli, CM; Furie, KL; et al. Pioglitazone after ischemic stroke or transient ischemic attack. *N Engl J Med*, 2016, 374(14), 1321-31.
[29] Tuccori, M; Filion, KB; Yin, H; et al., Pioglitazone use and risk of bladder cancer: Population based cohort study. *BMJ*, 2016, 352, i1541.

[30] Lewis, JD; Habel, LA; Quesenberry, CP; et al. Pioglitazone use and risk of bladder cancer and other common cancers in persons with diabetes. *JAMA*, 2015, 314, 265-77.

[31] Pop, LM; Lingvay, I; Yuan, Q; et al. Impact of pioglitazone on bone mineral density and bone marrow fat content. *Osteoporos Int*, 2017, 28, 3261-9.

[32] Lavine, JE; Schwimmer, JB; van Natta, ML; et al. Effect of vitamin E or metformin for treatment of nonalcoholic fatty liver disease in children and adolescents: The TONIC randomized controlled trial. *JAMA*, 2011, 305, 1659-68.

[33] Kowdley, KV; Van Natta, ML; Pai, RK, et al. Abstract 107: Efficacy and safety of vitamin E in nonalcoholic steatohepatitis patients with and without diabetes: Pooled analysis from the PIVENS and FLINT NIDDK NASH CRN Trials, *Hepatology*, 2015, 62(1Suppl), 264A.

[34] Miller, ER; Pastor-Barriuso, R; Dalal, D; et al. Meta-analysis: high-dosage vitamin E supplementation may increase all-cause mortality. *Ann Int Med*, 2005, 142(1), 37-46.

[35] Klein, EA; Thompson, IM; Jr. Tangen, CM; et al. Vitamin E and the risk of prostate cancer: The Selenium and Vitamin E Cancer Prevention Trial (SELECT). *JAMA*, 2011, 306, 1549-56.

[36] Dietrich, M; Jacques, PF; Pencina, MJ; et al. Vitamin E supplement use and the incidence of cardiovascular disease and all-cause mortality in the Framingham Heart Study: Does the underlying health status play a role? *Atherosclerosis*, 2009, 205, 549-53.

[37] Armstrong, MJ; Gaunt, P; Aithal, GP; et al. Liraglutide safety and efficacy in patients with non-alcoholic steatohepatitis (LEAN): A multicentre, double-blind, randomized, placebo-controlled phase 2 study. *Lancet*, 2016, 387, 679-90.

[38] Zeng, T; Zhang, CL; Zhao, XL; et al. Pentoxifylline for the treatment of nonalcoholic fatty liver disease: A meta-analysis of randomized double-blind, placebo-controlled studies. *Eur J Gastroenterol Hepatol*, 2014, 26, 646-53.

[39] Rakoski, MO; Singal, AG; Rogers, MA; et al. Meta-analysis: Insulin sensitizers for the treatment of non-alcoholic steatohepatitis. *Aliment Pharmacol Ther*, 2010, 32, 1211-21.

[40] Leuschner, UF; Lindenthal, B; Herrmann, G; et al. High-dose ursodeoxycholic acid therapy for nonalcoholic steatohepatitis: Adouble-blind, randomized, placebo-controlled trial. *Hepatology*, 2010, 52, 472-9.

[41] Musso, G; Gambino, R; Cassader, M; et al. A meta-analysis of randomized trials for the treatment of nonalcoholic fatty liver disease. *Hepatology*, 2010, 52, 79-104.

[42] Dasarathy, S; Dasarathy, J; Khiyami, A; et al. Double-blind randomized placebo-controlled clinical trial of omega 3 fatty acids for the treatment of diabetic patients with nonalcoholic steatohepatitis. *J Clin Gastroenterol*, 2015, 49, 137-44.

[43] Fernandez-Miranda, C; Perez-Carreras, M; Colina, F; et al. A pilot trial of fenofibrate for the treatment of non-alcoholic fatty liver disease. *Dig Liver Dis*., 2008, 40, 200-5.

[44] Basaranoglu, M; Acbay, O; Sonsuz, A. A controlled trial of gemfibrozil in the treatment of patients with non-alcoholic steatohepatitis. *J Hepatol*, 1999, 31, 384.

[45] Neuschwander-Tetri, BA; Loomba, R; Sanyal, AJ; et al. Farnesoid X nuclear receptor ligand obeticholic acid for non cirrhotic, non-alcoholic steatohepatitis (FLINT). A multicentre, randomized, placebo-controlled trial. *Lancet*, 2015, 385, 956-65.

[46] Friedman, S; Sanyal, A; Goodman, Z; et al. Efficacy and safety study of cenicriviroc for the treatment of non-alcoholic steatohepatitis in adult subjects with liver fibrosis: CENTAUR phase 2b study design. *Contemp Clin Trials*, 2016, 47, 356-65.

[47] Ratziu, V; Harrison, SA; Francque, S; et al. Elafibranor, an agonist of the peroxisome proliferator-activated receptor alpha and delta, induces resolution of nonalcoholic steatohepatitis without fibrosis worsening. *Gastroenterology*, 2016, 150, 1147-59, e5.

[48] Loomba, R; Lawitz, E; Mantry, PS; et al. The ASK1 inhibitor selonsertib in patients with nonalcoholic steatohepatitis: A randomized, phase 2 trial. *Hepatology.*, 2017, 67(2), 549-59.

[49] Lawitz, E; et al. Proof of concept study of an apoptosis-signal regulating kinase (ASK1) inhibitor (selonsertib) in combination with an acetyl-CoA carboxylase inhibitor (GS-0976) or a farnesoid X receptor agonist (GS-9674) in NASH. *J Hepathology*, 2018, 68, S57.

[50] Clinical Trials. gov. Safety and Efficacy of Selonsertib in Adults With Compensated Cirrhosis Due to Nonalcoholic Steatohepatitis (NASH) (STELLAR 4).

[51] Clinical Trials.gov. Emricasan, a Caspase inhibitor, for evaluation in subjects with non-alcoholic steatohepatitis (NASH) Fibrosis (ENCORENF), https://clinicaltrials.gov/ct2/show/NCT02686762.

[52] Safadi, R; Konikoff, FM; Mahamid, M; et al. The fatty acid-bile acid conjugate Aramchol reduces liver fat content in patients with nonalcoholic fatty liver disease. *Clin Gastroenterol Hepatol*, 2014, 12, 2085-91.

[53] Clinical Trials.gov. A Clinical Trial to Evaluate the Efficacy and Safety of Two Aramchol Doses Versus Placebo in Patients With NASH, https://clinicaltrials.gov/ct2/show/NCT02279524.

[54] Loomba, R; Lawitz, E; Parvez, S; et al. GS-4997, an Inhibitor of Apoptosis Signal-Regulating Kinase (ASK1), Alone or in Combination with Simtu-zumab for the Treatment of Nonalcoholic Steatohepatitis (NASH): A Randomized, Phase 2 Trial. *Hepatology*, 2016, 64(6), Suppl. 119A-120.

[55] Harrison, SA; Torgerson, S; Hayashi, P; et al. Vitamine E and vitamine C treatment improves fibrosis in patients with nonalcoholic steatohepatitis. *Am Gastroenterol*, 2003, 98(11), 2485-90.

[56] Okura, Y; Namisaki, T; Moriya, K; et al. Combined treatment with dipeptidyl peptidase-4 inhibitor (sitagliptin) and angiotensin-II type 1 receptor blocker (losartan) suppresses progression in a non-diabetic rat model of steatohepatitis. *Hepatol Res*, 2017, (47), 12, 1317-28.

ABOUT THE EDITORS

Jaime Ruiz-Tovar

Professor, Department of Surgery; Bariatric Surgery Unit,
Hospital Rey Juan Carlos University, Madrid, Spain

Jaime Ruiz-Tovar, MD, PhD is the Head of the Neurostimulation Unit at Garcilaso Clinic (Madrid, Spain), Bariatric Surgeon at Centro de Excelencia para el Tratamiento de la Obesidad (Valladolid, Spain), and Rey Juan Carlos University Hospital (Madrid, Spain). He is a Professor of Surgery, at the Universidad Alfonso X (Madrid, Spain). Dr. Tovar is the Head of the ERAS-Spain group in Bariatric Surgery, as well as the author of 11 books and multiple articles in scientific journals about obesity and bariatric surgery.

Lorea Zubiaga

Post-Doc, Lille University, Inserm-UMR.1190 – EGID/Lille, France

Lorea Zubiaga, MD, PhD is a digestive and general surgeon trained in bariatric surgery under the SECO-System (Spanish Society for Obesity and Metabolic Diseases). She dedicated her scientific thesis to unraveling the mechanisms of action of metabolic surgery. She is currently postdoctoral researcher at the European Genomic Institute for Diabetes (EGID) in Lille

(France) at the INSERM- UMR.1190 (Translational Research Laboratory for Diabetes -TRLD-). This unit mainly develops research projects related to the surgical treatment of type 1 diabetes (Langerhans islets transplant) and type 2 diabetes (metabolic surgery). The TRLD is also involved in different studies on obesity and liver steatosis. Dr. Zubiaga has published different articles in scientific journals and has been speaker in several national and international events.

INDEX

A

B

C

D

E

F

G

H

I

K

L

M

N

O

P

T

U

V

Related Nova Publications

Handbook of Surgical Procedures

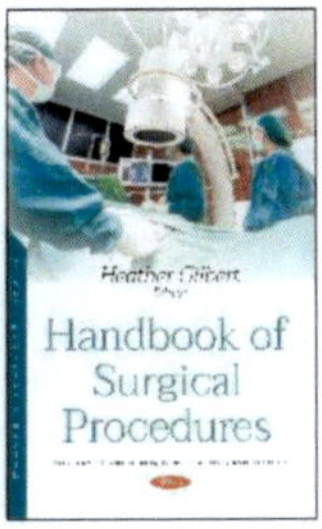

Editor: Heather Gilbert

Series: Surgery – Procedures, Complications, and Results

Book Description: In this compilation, the authors begin with a focus on the indications for surgery in hepatocarcinoma and how to perform a liver resection. Long-term outcomes and different theories on the causes of recurrence after resection are also discussed.

Hardcover ISBN: 978-1-53614-580-9
Retail Price: $128

Robotic Surgery: Clinical Perceptions, Approaches and Challenges

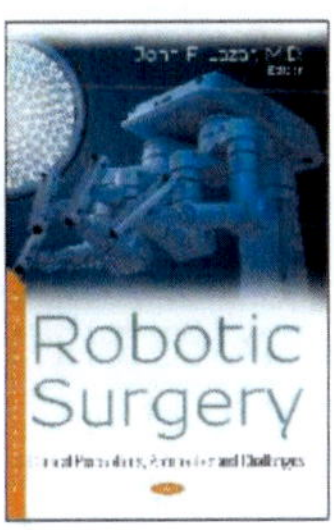

Editor: John F. Lazar, M.D.

Series: Robotics Research and Technology

Book Description: Robotic surgery is at a significant intersection of technology and the ability to routinely perform high-end minimal invasive surgery. *Robotic Surgery: Clinical Perceptions, Approaches and Challenges* is the robotic surgeon's manual to help achieve the technical and intellectual metrics desired by all surgeons.

Hardcover ISBN: 978-1-53614-325-6
Retail Price: $230

To see a complete list of Nova publications, please visit our website at www.novapublishers.com